T0280148

Health Care for Refugees and Displaced People

Catherine Mears and Sue Chowdhury

Oxfam
UK and Ireland

First published by Oxfam UK and Ireland in 1994
Reprinted in 1995, 2000, 2001, 2002, 2003

This version transferred to print-on-demand in 2006

© Oxfam UK and Ireland 1994

ISBN 0 85598 225 X

A catalogue record for this publication is available from the British Library.

Available from:

Bournemouth English Book Centre, PO Box 1496, Parkstone, Dorset, BH12 3YD, UK
tel: +44 (0)1202 712933; fax: +44 (0)1202 712930; email: oxfam@bebc.co.uk

USA: Stylus Publishing LLC, PO Box 605, Herndon, VA 20172-0605, USA
tel: +1 (0)703 661 1581; fax: +1 (0)703 661 1547; email: styluspub@aol.com

For details of local agents and representatives in other countries, consult our website:
www.oxfam.org.uk/publications
or contact Oxfam Publishing, Oxfam House, John Smith Drive, Cowley, Oxford,
OX4 2JY, UK
tel +44 (0) 1865 473727; fax (0) 1865 472393; email: publish@oxfam.org.uk

Our website contains a fully searchable database of all our titles, and facilities for secure
on-line ordering.

Published by Oxfam GB, Oxfam House, John Smith Drive, Cowley, Oxford, OX4 2JY, UK

Oxfam GB is a registered charity, no. 202918, and is a member of Oxfam International.

Contents

Acknowledgements   vii

Introduction   1

1 Assessment and planning   3
1.1 Introduction   3
1.2 Checklist of information required for assessment   5
    1.2.1 Demography   5
    1.2.2 Camp environment   5
    1.2.3 Logistics   6
    1.2.4 Shelter   7
    1.2.5 Environmental health   7
        Water
        Sanitation and vector control
        Hygiene promotion
    1.2.6 Food and nutrition   9
        Nutritional status
        Food availability
        General ration
        Selective feeding
    1.2.7 Health status and medical care   11
        Mortality
        Morbidity
        Medical care
    1.2.8 Psycho-social issues   12
1.3 Planning   13
    1.3.1 Assessment as the basis for planning   13
    1.3.2 Operational principles   13
        Standardisation
        Integration
        Participation and co-ordination
        Appropriate level of services
        Equity and ease of access

Preventive and curative care
1.2.3 General issues   15

2 Implementation and monitoring   17
2.1 Health Information System   17
2.2 Food and nutrition   18
2.2.1 Nutritional status   18
2.2.2 General feeding   19
Purpose
Admission criteria
Discharge criteria
Content
Method of distribution
2.2.3 Supplementary feeding   20
Purpose
Admission criteria
Discharge criteria
Content
Method of distribution
2.2.4 Therapeutic feeding   22
Purpose
Admission criteria
Discharge criteria
Content
Method of distribution
2.2.5 Monitoring   23
Nutritional surveillance
General ration programme
Supplementary and therapeutic feeding
2.3 Preventive health care   24
2.3.1 Environmental Health   24
Water supply
Sanitation and waste disposal
Vector control
Shelter
2.3.2 Immunisation   29
2.3.3 Health promotion   31
2.4 Control of communicable diseases   31

2.4.1 Summary of main methods for controlling diseases   32
2.4.2 Investigating disease outbreaks (epidemics)   32
2.4.3 Control of common diseases   33
   Measles
   Diarrhoeal diseases
   Bacillary dysentery
   Malaria
   Acute respiratory infections
   Hepatitis
   Meningococcal meningitis
   Tuberculosis
   HIV/AIDS
2.5 Clinical Care   38
2.5.1 Physical facilities, structures, staffing   38
   Organisation of health centre
   Staffing
   Monitoring
2.5.2 Health care for women and children   41
2.5.3 Laboratory facilities   42
2.5.4 Essential drugs and equipment   42
   Drug procurement
2.6 Psychosocial issues   43
2.6.1 Identification of vulnerable groups   43
2.6.2 Rehabilitation: strengthening community coping mechanisms   44
2.6.3 Training in awareness of psychosocial issues   44
2.6.4 Post-traumatic stress disorder   45
2.6.5 Monitoring   45
2.7 Training   45
2.7.1 Training needs   46
2.7.2 Training issues   46
2.7.3 Training method   46

3 Issues arising from long-term displacement   48
3.1 Introduction   48
3.2 Health Information System   49
3.3 Nutrition   49
3.3.1 Food rations   50
3.3.2 Supplementary feeding programmes   50
3.4 Environmental health   50

3.5 Immunisation   51

3.6 Health promotion   51

3.7 Disease control   51

3.8 Disability   51

3.9 Clinical care   52

3.10 Psycho-social issues   52

3.11 Training   52

4 Evaluation   54

4.1 Purpose of evaluation   54

4.2 Timing and scope of evaluation   54

4.3 Information required for evaluation   54

4.4 Types of indicator   55

4.5 Data collection for evaluation   56

4.6 Participatory evaluation   56

4.7 Reporting and using the findings   57

Appendices

1 Mortality rates   59

2 Nutrition surveys   61

3 Nutritional values of food aid commodities   74

4 Vitamin and mineral deficiencies   76

5 Supplementary feeding recipes   82

6 Water quality and chlorination   87

7 Lists of essential drugs (basic and supplementary kits)   88

8 Treatment protocols for diarrhoea, fever (and chloroquine-resistant malaria), acute respiratory infections   92

9 Vaccine storage, immunisation schedules, drug storage   100

10 Sample monitoring and surveillance form   102

References and further reading   104

Glossary   106

Index   109

Acknowledgements

This book is a successor to Oxfam's *Practical Guide to Refugee Health Care*, first published in 1983; a book which proved to be extremely useful to a wide range of practitioners. In preparing this new book on the subject, we have tried to reflect experience over the intervening years, and to take account of comments from users; but we also wish to acknowledge our debt to the valuable work of Dr Paul Shears and Dr Tim Lusty, who produced the earlier book at a time when there were few other texts specifically addressing refugee issues.

We would like to thank our colleagues in Oxfam who kindly read and commented on early drafts. We extend thanks also to Dr Helen Young and Dr Derek Summerfield for their contributions, and in particular to Patricia Diskett and Dr Mike Toole for their very valuable comments on the final draft.

We have consulted many different sources while writing this book, and these are included in the list of references and further reading. However, we take full responsibility for any statements made or conclusions drawn in the present text.

Catherine Mears
Sue Chowdhury

Oxford, February 1994

Introduction

This book has been written to assist health workers in relief and refugee programmes. It is by no means a comprehensive textbook, nor an exhaustive 'how to do it'. It is intended as a reference tool for health workers with limited or no experience of emergency situations, to be used in conjunction with other texts and specialised guidelines, some of which are listed as Further Reading. It does not deal with immediate medical and surgical care, but with the health needs and priorities of people who have been forced to flee from their homes for whatever reasons. Many aid agencies are involved in programmes to help people remain in their homes through periods of food scarcity or other hardship. While this is clearly the best option, such interventions are not always possible or effective, especially in situations of armed conflict.

The term 'refugee' will be used loosely throughout the text to refer to all people who have fled from their homes, and have to live in camps or similar situations. Strictly speaking, 'refugees' are people who have fled across international borders to a host country, whereas 'displaced people' have also left their homes, but remain within their own country. The United Nations High Commissioner for Refugees (UNHCR) provides material assistance to refugees, at the request of host governments; displaced people do not normally receive such assistance. Displaced people may be worse off in other respects, especially if they have fled from violence associated with civil war, and have to live among fellow nationals who are hostile to them. Non-government agencies do not operate under the same restrictions as UNHCR and do assist displaced people in need wherever possible, as well as refugees. The International Committee of the Red Cross (ICRC), under the Geneva Convention, plays a special role in conflict areas, by providing protection and material assistance, including health care.

This book refers, for the most part, to the context of a refugee camp. However, many displaced people and refugees live dispersed in the settlements and towns of host populations, sometimes with relations or friends. While their health is often less endangered than that of people living in camps, the additional strain on family food supplies, sanitary conditions, and water supply may compromise their health

1

and perhaps that of their hosts. Camps can vary in size from a few dozen people to tens of thousands; and living quarters can range from flimsy, temporary shelters to permanent buildings. In this book, 'camp' refers to a large camp, or a grouping of smaller camps each with a population of around 10,000 or more.

While circumstances sometimes allow sites and shelters to be prepared before refugees arrive in the area, it is far more usual that health and other aid workers begin work in crowded, semi-established camps, with inadequate food, water supply, and shelter, indiscriminate 'non-sanitation', perhaps with a measles epidemic, and with most children apparently suffering from diarrhoea and pneumonia.

But even in the often distressing surroundings of a refugee camp, where needs may seem obvious, it is essential to plan and prioritise interventions with care, so that limited resources are used to the greatest effect. It has been shown that mortality and morbidity are reduced most effectively by providing adequate water and sanitation, uncrowded shelter, an adequate food supply, and organising a measles immunisation programme at an early stage. However, if there is widespread malnutrition, perhaps compounded by a diarrhoea epidemic, many people, especially young children, will only survive if they receive appropriate and timely medical care.

The book is divided into four sections. The first two, *Assessment and planning* and *Implementation and monitoring* deal with health issues most likely to arise in the first months after displacement, although, depending oncircumstances, this acute phase may last for up to a year. Unfortunately, many refugee situations are not resolved for many years, and the result is long-term settlement of impoverished outsiders in locations which are often unsuitable; and this will bring its own problems. The third section therefore gives a brief outline of *Issues arising from long-term displacement*, followed by a short section on *Evaluation*. Additional information is given in the technical appendices and glossary, and there is a list of useful and readily available sources for further reference.

1 Assessment and planning

1.1 Introduction

Speed is an important factor in deciding on the methods to be employed for an assessment. Depending on road conditions, size of camp area, number of refugees, and other factors, an assessment could take from a few days to as long as two weeks. It may include a nutrition survey, which can be combined with an attempt to quantify other public health problems, such as the incidence of diarrhoea. Appropriate methodologies include observation, interviews with key informants, particularly refugees, rapid nutritional assessments, and analysis of clinic data and similar documentation. Reports from other agencies or government sources may already be available. They should be used wherever possible, but should be interpreted with care, and some professional judgement may be required as to their reliability.

Assessment is essential to enable:

- an initial decision to be made on whether assistance is needed at all;
- a decision to be made on whether local capacity is adequate or external resources are required;
- priorities for intervention to be established, and a strategy for intervention identified;
- the collection of base-line data to facilitate monitoring.

Assessment must cover the following three areas:

1 The health and nutritional status of the refugees, which will depend both on the history of their displacement and conditions in the camp.
2 The risk factors in the camp environment, principally inadequate food, inadequate water and sanitation, inadequate and crowded shelter, and susceptibility to measles and other communicable diseases.
3 The local health resources, to identify gaps between existing resources and resource requirements. Both physical infrastructure and human resources,

3

including trained health workers among the refugees, should be assessed, and the availability of additional national and international health resources.

The assessment team should include people with the specialist skills to assess local epidemiological profile and health service capacity, and the health and nutritional status of the refugees, and to interpret the findings.

Worldwide, women and children constitute the majority of refugees, because men are often more mobile and leave in search of jobs or, in situations of armed conflict, to take part in the fighting. There may also be a disproportionate number of other vulnerable people in a camp, such as old people or people with disabilities. Security and protection are therefore especially important. Women may have been traumatised by violence and rape, especially those who have fled from areas of conflict. It is important that health services for refugees are particularly sensitive to the special health needs of women.

It is also advisable to disaggregate information about children by sex. Many societies discriminate in favour of male children, so that, for example, an overall acceptable level of malnutrition may hide a substantially higher proportion of malnourished girls. Similarly, sick girls are less likely to be taken to receive medical care than boys. During the assessment, it is therefore advisable to consider and refer to 'men' and 'women' rather than adults, and about 'boys' and 'girls' rather than children.

In the medium to longer term, or as soon as the situation has stabilised, anthropological, sociological, and general development methodologies should be integrated into the health assessment. A better understanding of the health behaviour and recent history of the people concerned should result in more appropriate health care and make it possible to address sensitive issues like psycho-social problems. During the initial assessment, when death rates may be high and the refugee population suffering extreme degrees of material deprivation, these methods may be difficult to apply because they usually take more time and rely on a degree of stability.

The following checklist is intended to serve as a reminder for the information which should be gathered during the assessment. It may not be feasible to answer all the questions in full but they serve as prompts and reminders of significant issues. All the questions on the checklist are related to the three principal components of health assessment identified above: health and nutrition status, major risk factors, and resource availability and requirements.

The questions in the checklist are grouped as follows: demography, camp environment, logistics, shelter, environmental health, food and nutrition, health status and medical care, psycho-social issues.

1.2 Checklist of information required for assessment

1.2.1 Demography

How many people are arriving, leaving, reported to be on the way, expected to arrive within the next days, weeks, or months?

How have these numbers been collected, or estimated?

Has a sample survey of shelters been carried out, to ascertain average household size?

Has a simple map of the camp been prepared?

What proportion of the camp population are men, women, boys, girls, and what proportion of children are under and what proportion over five years old?

What proportion are pregnant women, unaccompanied minors, elderly?

Is data on mortality available? Is it possible to calculate a daily rate?

1.2.2 Camp environment

Where have the refugees come from? Did they flee from armed conflict?

How long have they been on the way, and what conditions have they faced on their journey to the camp?

How far from the border are the refugees?

Are there any security problems around or inside the camp?

Do the refugees have any provisions, and were they able to bring any possessions with them?

What is the general situation with respect to food availability; health; and health services in the surrounding area?

What is the attitude of local leaders and communities to the new arrivals?

What is the terrain of the camp (desert plain, mountainous, swampy)?

Is the site planned or *ad hoc*? If it was planned, who was responsible?

What is the current season (rainy, dry, cold, hot) and what change is to be expected?

How is the camp being administered (if at all)? Is the local government involved? Are there refugee camp committees? Are local or international agencies involved?

Are women involved in camp administration?

Is there co-ordination between agencies, and if so, is it structured or *ad hoc*? Who is responsible for co-ordination? Is there any duplication of activities or funding?

1.2.3 Logistics

Transport

Are there all-weather roads to the site(s)? Is there access by air, river, or sea?

What is the source of available transport (private, government, military, agency)?

What facilities exist for servicing of and supplying fuel for vehicles?

Is there any problem of security of food deliveries?

Communications

How is contact made with the capital or nearest government centre, and is it reliable?

Is an agency communication system needed, or are local facilities available?

Is radio equipment required, and if so, is it permitted?

Storage

What storage facilities exist, and of what capacity?

Are the storage facilities secure, and how are they administered?

What is the level of hygiene for food stores?

Are the food stores weatherproof?

Staffing

What skills are available amongst the refugees and the local population?

How are skilled refugees identified and recruited?

Do workers receive salaries, incentives, or food for work?

What NGOs are active and what is the general level of their staffing, training, and funding capacity?

Money

What are the facilities for banking, money changing, and bartering?

1.2.4 Shelter

Materials

What sort of housing are the refugees accustomed to, and are the materials available locally for building it?

Are there any constraints to obtaining material locally (security of access, deforestation)?

Do materials available for housing allow for shade, protection from rain, and privacy?

Capacity

Are the shelters over-crowded? What is the average number of refugees per shelter?

Are families living separately or in groups?

Are there separate facilities for men and women?

Are cooking facilities separate from living areas?

Is there room for people to store their possessions and stocks of food?

Safety

What is the average distance between shelters?

Is there a high risk of fire, flooding, subsidence, landslips?

1.2.5 Environmental health

Water

How is water supplied to the population (standpipe, tanker)?

What is the source of water (river, well, cistern, rain)?

Is the source relatively clean and likely to remain so?

Is the source adequate in all seasons?

How close is the supply to the refugees' shelters?

What (approximately) is the consumption rate of water per head?

Is there evidence of a severe water-related disease problem (skin disease, typhoid, diarrhoea)?

Is there any danger of the source being contaminated from latrines, livestock or (in the case of rivers) other camps and settlements upstream?

Is there any danger of contamination to settlements downstream?

Is the water tested regularly? Is it tested at source, during distribution, or at household level?

Is there any system of water treatment?

If a pump is used, how is it serviced and what contingency plans are there if it breaks down?

Are washing facilities provided? Is so, where, and is there privacy for women?

Where are animals watered?

How is water stored in refugees' shelters? What containers are used for storage, and are they clean and covered?

Sanitation and vector control

Is there evidence of a high incidence of disease which could be related to excreta disposal (diarrhoea, worms)?

What is the normal practice of defecation of the refugee population (note that women's practices may be different from men's)?

How are excreta disposed of (family or communal system, pit latrines, water-borne system, cartage, random)? Is there a designated defecation area?

Is there sufficient space to allow for pit latrines to be dug?

Is water available for handwashing close to the defecation area?

How close is the water source to the sewage disposal point?

Is there an obvious problem with flies, rodents, cockroaches, mosquitoes, fleas, lice, or bedbugs?

How is solid waste and rubbish disposed of (collection system, burning, burial)?

Is the water table high or low?

What is the soil structure (rocky, sandy)?

How will different seasons affect existing sanitation systems (flooding)?

How is waste water drained off the site? Are there pools of standing water?

Hygiene promotion

What are the accepted beliefs and practices among the refugees? Are there cultural sensitivities, or taboo subjects?

Do the refugees understand the relationship between water, sanitation, shelter, vectors, and disease?

Do the refugees have previous experience of communal living?

What are the common hygiene practices among the refugees (washing hands after defecation, storage and covering of cooked food, disposal of children's faeces)?

Is hygiene promotion integrated both with technical work on water and sanitation and also with the health services?

1.2.6 Food and nutrition

Nutritional status

What major changes to their normal diet have occurred since the refugees left their homes or arrived in the camp?

What is the general impression of the nutritional situation? Do more than two in ten children appear very thin or wasted?

Are there children with evident oedema?

What anecdotal information is there about deaths from malnutrition?

Has a nutritional (anthropometric) survey been undertaken, and what were the findings? If not, are there plans to carry out a survey?

Are newcomers in better or worse condition than those already in the camp, or about the same?

Is there any evidence of specific nutritional deficiencies (vitamin A, B and C deficiency, iron-deficiency anaemia)?

Food availability

What foods are in short supply and is this expected to change?

What foods do refugees obtain locally through purchase or bartering?

Has the availability and price of foods in local markets altered recently? If so, how has this affected local people and refugees?

General ration

Has a general ration been agreed? What is the content of the food basket, and the daily energy value?

In practice, how regular is the distribution?

Are refugees actually receiving the agreed ration?

How is the distribution system organised? Who distributes the food, how often, to whom, what records are kept, and how orderly is the distribution?

In practice, how fair is the food distribution? Is any group excluded? How dowomen gain access?

Is cereal given milled or whole? Are milling facilities available?

What fuel for cooking, shelter for cooking, and cooking pots are available?

What opportunities are there for bartering items in the food basket?

Selective feeding: supplementary and therapeutic

What amount has been agreed, and by whom, for distribution as supplementary food (type of foods, daily energy and protein value)? In practice, are these foods regularly available?

How is it distributed? As part of the general ration, or in selective wet or dry feeding programmes?

What are the admission and discharge criteria for supplementary feeding?

Are pregnant and lactating women and severely malnourished adults admitted?

What records are kept? How regular is attendance of individual children at wet feeding centres?

What is the coverage of the supplementary feeding programme in relation to numbers malnourished (from surveys and screenings)?

Do people receive the full general ration that has been agreed, or is the supplementary food used as a substitute for an inadequate general ration?

If the wet feeding centre clean and well-organised? How is selective feeding linked with medical screening?

What nutritional and medical treatment is available for severely malnourished children?

Is vitamin A being routinely distributed?

1.2.7 Health status and medical care

Mortality

How is mortality being recorded? What is the extent of under-reporting?

Is there a designated burial area?

What is the crude mortality rate and under-five mortality rate (number of deaths per 10,000 people per day)?

What is the main cause of death?

In what age group are most deaths occurring?

Morbidity

How are the incidence and prevalence of diseases measured and recorded? Is there a standardised system? How is data analysed and used?

What are the main health problems in the camp? Which group, according to age and sex, is most affected? Is there a high incidence of communicable diseases such as diarrhoea, malaria, or acute respiratory infection?

What are the major camp risk factors (inadequate water and sanitation facilities, crowding, inadequate food)?

Are there cases of measles, and how are these monitored?

What is the rate of acute malnutrition, how is this monitored?

Are there cases of micronutrient deficiency disorders, and how are these monitored?

Are there cases of dysentery, and how are these monitored?

Is the camp in a malaria-endemic area? Are there cases of malaria, and how are these monitored?

Are there specific health problems for women (high birth rate, anaemia, sexually transmitted diseases)?

Medical care

What health infrastructure exists locally, including referral capacity?

Who manages the health care system in the camp?

How are resources for health care (material and human) distributed?

How much refugee participation is there (health committees)? Are refugees involved in decisions about health provision?

Are simple preventive measures being taken to reduce risk factors for communicable diseases?

Is measles immunisation taking place? What are the coverage rates?

Is there an effective cold chain?

Is there a facility for oral rehydration therapy?

Is there a sufficient supply of ORS?

Are any health promotion activities being organised?

Are there health centres or health posts already built in the camp? What medical equipment is available?

Are repairs to existing facilities or new construction required?

Are there special health facilities available for women and children?

Are essential drugs available and are standardised case definitions and prescribing and treatment protocols being followed?

What health personnel are available and what is their level of training and competence? Are there female health workers?

How are the health workers paid?

What training and supervisory systems for health workers have been organised?

Is there a system of triage of outpatients to identify the most seriously ill?

Is there a referral system for health problems which the camp medical facilities are unable to deal with?

1.2.8 Psycho-social issues

Were the refugees forced to leave their homes suddenly, under threat of violence?

Did the refugees suffer days, weeks or months of lack of food, water, security?

Is there still a continuing threat of violence or harassment in the camp (factional fighting, gunfire, rape, intimidation, abductions)?

What is the extent of bereavement (dead or missing relatives) and loss: loss of livelihood, personal possessions, privacy, social status, social cohesion, dignity (standing in queues, handouts)?

What is the extent of cultural bereavement i.e. loss of 'home' in the widest sense, including a surrounding landscape as the repository of origin myths, religious symbolism, and history?

Do refugees have personal histories of torture, witnessing atrocities, or being forced to participate in atrocities?

Do the refugees constitute a fragmented community, with mixed ethnic, religious, and political factions?

Is there a lack of employment opportunities, boredom, a 'temporary-permanent-transit' status in the camp?

What are the health beliefs and traditions of the refugees?

1.3 Planning

The aim of a refugee health programme is to reduce mortality and morbidity and to maintain them at as low a level as possible. Well-defined health policies with explicit aims and objectives form the basis of planning.

1.3.1 Assessment as the basis for planning
The information collected during the assessment will have clarified the scale of the situation, including the severity of the crisis, the number of people affected, and their actual and projected needs. This information will enable detailed plans to be made. It is useful to begin by summarising the data and listing the problems to be tackled in order of importance. Objectives can then be formulated, priorities for intervention identified, indicators selected for monitoring and evaluation, and a plan of action worked out. The plan must have a realistic budget attached to it. Whilst food and other relief items are often donated, staff salaries are usually a major part of the overall cost to the implementing agency.

Speed with clarity is essential, because in the early stages the situation is likely to be dynamic and confusing for all involved.

1.3.2 Operational principles
Planning should be guided by some essential operational principles:

Standardisation
Working methods, equipment and drug lists should be coordinated and agreed

between all parties, including local health authorities and other government agencies, refugee representatives, and non-governmental organisations. Usually Ministries of Health and UN agencies have developed standard guidelines for the provision of health care. These should be respected and adopted wherever possible.

Integration

Services should be integrated so that whenever feasible they are available from the same fixed site(s) and managed as part of a comprehensive service. Integrated programmes are usually more appropriate and sustainable than programmes which have separate management structures and resources ('vertical' programmes), though such programmes may be necessary for specific emergency interventions such as measles immunisation or supplementary feeding. In large camps, facilities should be decentralised to improve access.

Participation and co-ordination

Refugees should always be consulted in the planning of any measures or services affecting them. In particular, it is essential that the concerns of refugee women are listened to and taken into account. Women should be consulted to ensure that services are accessible to them and appropriate to their needs.

Services for refugees should be co-ordinated with the health structures in the host country and community, with other government agencies, multilateral and non-governmental organisations who are working in the camps, and with refugee representatives. If appropriate, specific responsibilities should be assigned to different agencies. Parallel structures should be avoided as far as possible. Clear lines of responsibility for health co-ordination should be established.

Appropriate level of services

The health of the refugees depends on all the measures taken which help to reduce camp risk factors, most notably inadequate food supply, crowding, and inadequate water and sanitation, and also on basic preventive and curative health care, i.e. a 'primary health care' approach.

The main elements of the health-care system should be preventive care and health promotion, basic curative care, and monitoring and surveillance. Those in need of secondary medical care are usually referred to health centres or hospitals outside the camp, if available. These referral facilities should have been identified during the assessment of the local health infrastructure.

The system will require a physical infrastructure: basic health posts and possibly health centres depending on resources, population size, and host country facilities. It may also be necessary to provide separate centres for selective feeding.

Health care staff will need to be identified. Local expertise should be used whenever possible, and training, supervision and remuneration policies and procedures agreed between implementing agencies.

Equity and ease of access
The needs of all sections of the population should be considered. This may mean that special arrangements have to be made for vulnerable groups who may otherwise have limited or no access to health services. It is particularly important to make sure that services are accessible to women, to elderly and to disabled people, and to minority groups. Special arrangements may include flexible opening times of clinics, and the siting of facilities in secure areas. Steps should be taken to ensure that women are well represented among the health staff, and that the health needs of women are considered in thetraining of both male and female staff.

Preventive and curative care
Emphasis should be on the prevention of ill-health through improvements in environmental health, ensuring and monitoring food availability, providing adequate shelter, and health promotion. However, the management of existing health problems must also be addressed. Treatment of infected individuals may be a key element of disease control (e.g. malaria, see p.34).

1.3.3 General issues
Other general factors to consider at the planning stage are:

Resources
In the early stages of an emergency, particularly if there is a high media profile, donors usually provide adequate funds, but these may reduce substantially if the refugee situation is prolonged. Planning should allow for this.

Logistics
Reliable supplies of equipment, spare parts, consumable items, and essential drugs will have to be organised. The functioning of a health programme will be seriously affected by erratic supply.

Communal relations
Problems often arise between the refugees and the host community, and every effort should be made to foster good relations. This will depend partly on a clear assessment of the socio-political situation in the affected areas, and the capacity and orientation of existing NGOs and UN agencies.

Refugees often use local health facilities, especially if they are referred for secondary medical care. Resources should be set aside to strengthen local health services to cope with the additional workload and demands on resources. UNHCR has a 'refugee affected area' policy (sometimes called the 'cross-mandate policy') which provides for this. In addition, camp resources and facilities, such as feeding centres, can be made accessible to local people if there is a need.

2 Implementation and monitoring

2.1 Health Information System (HIS)

The assessment data form the basis for initial decisions and planning of the response. The method of recording and communicating information about the existing health status of a population is known as a Health Information System (HIS). A HIS is needed to:

- follow trends and establish health care priorities;
- detect early evidence of outbreaks of disease, for immediate response;
- monitor effectiveness and coverage of the health-care programme;
- ensure that resources are targeted to areas of greatest need;
- evaluate the health programme;
- provide information for lobbying for more resources if necessary.

The two main sources of health information are data collected through clinic returns, and reports from community health workers and home visitors (passive surveillance); and data collected through periodic sample surveys and disease outbreak investigations (active surveillance). Anecdotal reports should also be given consideration.

There may already be a system in place, and there may be few if any changes required. It is nevertheless important to ensure that responsibilities for reporting and monitoring are clearly assigned. It is important that clear case definitions and treatment protocols have been established and agreed, and used by all health personnel (see Appendix 8). Health workers will need some training in data collection and use, and accurate recording. The use of simple forms, for clinic returns, house-to-house visits, and health promotion, can help in this task. The minimum routine action at health-centre level is to maintain a graph of disease incidence.

Data should be collected on:(see Appendices for more detail)

- deaths (related to age, sex and cause); **in the emergency phase, mortality is the most specific indicator of health status;**

17

- nutritional status;
- morbidity (rate, sex and age specific, cause);
- births;
- population movement, rate of arrivals and departures;
- sub-groups at special risk e.g. pregnant women, children under five, unaccompanied children;
- programme information (immunisations, feeding programmes, clinic attendance).

Data collection should be limited to information which can and will be acted upon. The data must then be collated, validated, analysed, interpreted, and fed back to the staff. This will usually be the responsibility of the medical co-ordinator in collaboration with the refugee administration and will be done through mechanisms such as co-ordination meetings, bulletins etc.

It is essential that all health workers are fully aware of how the data will be used and understand the importance of accurate data for the quality of their work.

Computerisation of health records may be considered, depending on the complexity of the programme, resources available, and technical capacity.

2.2 Food and nutrition

2.2.1 Nutritional status

To assess the nutritional status of refugees the rate (prevalence) of malnutrition is estimated by measuring a sample of children under five years of age. The weight-for-height index which reflects acute malnutrition (thinness or wasting) is the most common nutritional index used to assess short-term nutritional problems. Guidelines for a simple nutritional (anthropometric) survey are given in Appendix 2. (More detailed information can be found in Oxfam's Practical Health Guide No.7 (1992) *Food Scarcity and Famine: Assessment and Response.*)

A nutritional survey should be carried out as early as possible. During the emergency phase, surveys should be repeated at three- to six-monthly intervals. A survey indicates the severity of the nutritional situation, provides a baseline for monitoring, and information essential for planning purposes. Clear objectives for the survey should be defined. If the results are to be used to compare with other surveys, this has implications for sample size.

When a survey is carried out, recognised survey methods should always be used:

- standardised weighing and measuring techniques;
- nutritional indices (usually weight-for-height, given in Appendix 2);
- accepted reference values (usually WHO/NCHS/CDC international reference population, given in Appendix 2);
- reliable sampling methods.

Staff may need to be trained in the use of these techniques. It is also important that the purpose of the survey and the methods to be used are fully explained to refugees, and that the procedure is acceptable to them.

The results of different nutritional surveys should only be compared if similar methods have been used, otherwise you are not comparing like with like. When interpreting the results of nutritional surveys, it is important to consider the underlying causes of nutritional problems. High rates of wasting (acute malnutrition) may be the result of either an inadequate diet or outbreaks of infectious diseases, particularly measles. In a situation where children are exposed to high levels of communicable diseases, malnutrition is more dangerous than in a situation where health risks are few. Careful interpretation of results helps in deciding which interventions are needed most.

Interpretation of results

Interpretation of results involves comparison with nutritional status of the local population, consideration of the pre-flight characteristics of the refugees, and seasonal factors. As a rough guide, a global malnutrition rate of more than 10 per cent should suggest further investigation and intervention. (The malnutrition rate is the proportion with less than 80 per cent weight-for-height, and oedema, or the proportion of less than two standard deviations, and oedema; for more detail see Appendix 2.) A rate of 15 per cent and over suggests a critical situation.

A high rate of malnutrition not only means that many children are malnourished, but also that there are more children who could soon become malnourished should conditions deteriorate. However, a low rate can also mean that many of the most severely malnourished children have already died. Figures obtained from anthropometric surveys have therefore to be used in conjunction with figures for morbidity and mortality, in order to provide an accurate picture of the situation.

2.2.2 General feeding

Purpose

A general ration is intended to provide everybody with their nutritional requirements. The relief food ration should be calculated to take into account factors such as climatic conditions and refugees' access to alternative means of subsistence. Some rations consist of a staple food only, but this should only be given to refugees who have regular access to other sources of food.

Content

The 'food basket' usually consists of a staple food, such as sorghum, wheat or rice, plus a source of protein (beans or lentils), and a source of fat (oil). UNHCR and WFP have agreed this should provide a minimum of 1900 Kcal/person/day. In a balanced ration, protein should provide 12.5 per cent of total energy and fat should provide at least 10.0 per cent of total energy. A sample ration would be within the following ranges:-

weight gm	food	energy Kcal	protein gm	fat gm
350-500	cereal	1155-1650	35-55	7-8
20-40	oil	180-360	0	178-356
50-100	pulses	175-350	10-20	1-2

However, this food basket is not nutritionally balanced as it is deficient in essential vitamins and minerals, such as vitamin A, and vitamin C, which refugees must obtain from other sources if they are to avoid deficiency diseases. The general food basket should also contain a blended food such as Corn-Soy Blend (CSB) or Wheat-Soy Blend (WSB), for use by small children, the sick, and the malnourished. The blended food should be fortified with vitamins.

Method of distribution

Food should be distributed from fixed sites at regular intervals, say monthly. Often it is the family head who is registered and who then receives the ration on behalf of the family. It is preferable to distribute food rations to women, as they are normally responsible for procuring and preparing food. Also, in polygamous societies, this ensures each co-wife receives a share. Refugees themselves, especially women, should be involved in the distribution as much as possible. Distribution could, for example, be administered by a camp committee.

2.2.3 Supplementary feeding

Purpose

A supplementary feeding programme is set up to treat children who are moderately malnourished and to prevent severe malnutrition developing. Severely malnourished children may also be included if there is no separate therapeutic programme. The programme may also include the provision of a nutritious food supplement to pregnant and lactating women, and sick, and particularly vulnerable people (orphans, socially isolated, traumatised), if resources allow.

Supplementary feeding should be part of a larger health-care programme including immunisation, vitamin A supplementation, and the prevention and treatment of communicable diseases.

A feeding programme is indicated, for example, where the malnutrition rate is more than 15 per cent (less than 80 per cent weight-for-height); or the general ration is less than 1500 Kcals/person/day; or where the general ration is approximately 1900 Kcals/person/day but there are high rates of diarrhoea or measles.

Admission criteria
Recognised vulnerable groups such as moderately malnourished children (between 70 per cent and 80 per cent weight-for-height, or between Z-scores -2 and -3). In a situation where rates of acute malnutrition (less than 80 per cent weight-for-height or Z-score -2) are very high and there are severe health risks in the camp environment, it may be more appropriate to admit all children under a given age to supplementary feeding, if resources allow. This would prevent children who are just above the admission criteria level from deteriorating further.

Discharge criteria
A child is discharged when it has maintained a weight-for-height ratio of more than 85 per cent for one month (or a Z-score of -1.5).

Content
Supplementary rations should be nutritionally adequate as a weaning food for infants and for young children. They must be energy dense (rich in fat or oil), high in protein, and a good source of vitamins and minerals. They must also be palatable. The aim should be to provide approximately 500–800 kcal/person/day. In some situations a failure of the general ration may mean that people are getting less than 1900 kcal/person/day, in which case the supplementary ration may have to be increased to protect the most vulnerable in the short-term. However, this is not effective in the longer-term as a substitute for the full general ration.

High energy biscuits may be used in the initial stages of a supplementary feeding programme. They are readily available but are expensive to use in a long-term programme. They are useful for take-home rations and to boost calories in a milk or porridge mixture. They should only be used under supervision, not distributed widely.

Method of distribution
There are two methods of distribution, 'wet' and 'dry'. In wet distribution, food is cooked daily and eaten at a feeding centre. In dry distribution, uncooked foods are distributed to refugees to take home on a regular basis (weekly or two-weekly); the

size of the ration should be increased to allow for sharing with other children in the family. Generally, dry distribution is easier to manage, with those persistently failing to gain weight referred to the therapeutic feeding programme. Dry distribution usually improves uptake because it is less demanding of women's time. Large wet-feeding centres may increase disease transmission if poorly supervised. The maximum number of beneficiaries per centre should be 500.

2.2.4 Therapeutic feeding

Purpose
Therapeutic feeding programmes are intended to rehabilitate severely malnourished children and adults through intensive feeding of special foods, and health care.

Therapeutic feeding programmes require a high level of resources, in particular the time and expertise of health workers. Naso-gastric feeding may be necessary. Skilled and trained staff are essential. Severely malnourished children with medical complications have a high mortality risk, even where feeding and medical care is available.

Admission criteria
All children less that 70 per cent weight-for-height (or Z-score -3) and all children with kwashiorkor, should be admitted. Medical screening of admissions and regular medical supervision is vital. Loss of appetite is common; children need to be continuously coaxed and encouraged to eat. Malnourished adults may also need to be admitted, and also pregnant women with severe anaemia.

Discharge criteria
Children should be discharged to a supplementary feeding programme when they have maintained 80 per cent weight-for-height for at least two weeks, with no oedema and no medical problem.

Content
The foods given should be energy dense, high in protein, and a good source of vitamins and minerals, especially vitamin A. High-energy milk is commonly used, along with other recipes. For young children it should be liquid (high energy milk) or semi-liquid (porridge). A malnourished child needs a minimum of 150 kcal and 3 to 4g protein /kg body weight/ day.

Breastfeeding must continue. If breastfeeding is not possible, the child should be fed with a spoon and cup. Bottles and beakers should always be avoided because they are difficult to keep clean in the usual refugee camp environment.

Method of distribution
Through special feeding centres, which may be a 24-hour facility or daytime only. At least six or seven feeds should be provided throughout the day and night, rather than fewer larger feeds. The maximum number of patients per centre should be around 50.

2.2.5 Monitoring

Nutritional surveillance
Regular monitoring (every three months minimum in the emergency phase) of nutritional status should provide a sensitive indicator of the underlying health and nutrition situation. However, results should be carefully interpreted taking into account that acute malnutrition may be the result of inadequate food intake or disease, or both. Seasonal variation in nutritional status may also be significant.

Screening
As well as undertaking periodic sample surveys, all children under five years of age should undergo nutritional screening on arrival at the camp. MUAC (mid-upper arm circumference) is a useful screening method as it can be carried out quickly in order to select children who need further assessment (using weight-for-height) for admission to a feeding programme. MUAC may also be used for ongoing screening in child-health clinics and in the homes, by community health workers. See Appendix 2 for details.

General ration programme
Nutritional surveillance should indicate the incidence of malnutrition, and the emergence of new nutritional deficiencies, if any. The practical functioning of the distribution should also be monitored, looking at reliability (timing, and content of the ration basket), coverage, access, and security. The availability of other sources of food to which refugees have access, and their opportunities for earning income and bartering the ration should also be monitored.

Supplementary and therapeutic feeding
Monitoring of these programmes should consist of recording the weight gain of individual children, and assessing regularity of attendance, coverage (proportion of children included in the programme compared with the proportion malnourished), cases of death, and access to centres or distribution points.

2.3 Preventive health care

2.3.1 Environmental health

Clean water, adequate sanitation and rubbish disposal are essential for the health of the population. But purely technical interventions such as the construction of latrines, or the drilling of boreholes do not of themselves ensure a healthy environment. Hygiene promotion, together with these technical inputs, is an important component of environmental health work. Hygiene promotion helps to raise public awareness and influences hygiene practices at community, household, and individual level. This is particularly important where systems unfamiliar to the refugees are introduced.

Water supply

Most refugee camps are situated close to an existing ground or surface water supply. This may be insufficient in quantity and rapidly deteriorate in quality, as increasing numbers of people attempt to collect water. When improvement to the water supply is undertaken during the emergency phase, it is more important to increase quantity than to improve quality. There are many degrees of technical sophistication for improving water supplies, ranging from simple spring protection to the installation of high-tech equipment. Technically simple methods, which build on local systems and use local materials, are preferable, provided they supply adequate quantities of water for the refugees' needs. Acceptable standards of water quality are given in detail in Appendix 6 Seasonal variations may have an effect on water quantity and quality, and plans for water supply need to anticipate this.

Immediate action: Whatever water source people are using when you arrive at the site (river, lake, well) take immediate steps to protect that source and to prevent any further pollution. This could mean fencing off the water, moving people up river, or moving animals.

Technical inputs: If a water and sanitation engineer is not part of the initial assessment team and work is not already in progress to improve water supplies, the issue should be addressed urgently. It is highly likely that a technical input will be required. Remember that the choice of technology, and the system of maintenance and management, may be a political issue. Opt for basic systems first, then upgrade later.

Quantity of water required: For drinking purposes only, the absolute minimum requirement is 3 litres/person/day. More is usually required, amounts depending on level of activity and ambient temperature. For all purposes, including cooking, washing, laundry, approximately 15 litres/person/day is required. WHO/UNHCR recommend 20 litres/person/day but this may not be feasible. Try not to give less than 8 litres/person/day as an absolute minimum. If too little water is available, personal hygiene will be compromised and transmission of water-related diseases will increase.

There will also be requirements for the functioning of feeding centres (20-30 litres per patient per day) and health centres, where the amount required will depend on the activities.

Consultation: It is important to liaise with the local water authority and involve refugees, particularly women who are the collectors and main users of water

Carrying water: The aim should be to take water to the people, not people to the water. Try to keep water carrying distances down to a minimum. Most water is carried to the household by women, and sometimes by children. The distance of the water source from the shelter strongly influences the quantity of water used, due to the time and effort required to carry it, and sometimes to security risks.

It may be necessary to provide women with water collecting and storage containers such as plastic jerry cans. Lack of adequate containers will affect both quantity carried and quality.

Trucking or tankering water: Trucking water should be seen as a first, temporary measure not a medium- or long-term solution. There may be exceptional circumstances where no other option is available.

If it is suggested that water is brought in by tanker or storage tanks are to be prepared, basic calculations of quantity are essential. For all purposes 1000 litres will provide water for 66 people for one day. A water tanker of 8000 litres capacity will thus supply water for 530 people, or drinking water only for 2,700 people. If tankering is used, do not distribute direct from the tanker. Always off-load into a separate tank, and ensure a tap bar is attached.

Preventing pollution: A natural source may be rapidly polluted, both directly, by people crowding round streams and river beds, or less directly, by run-off rainfall spreading surface contamination into the source. Pollution can be dramatically reduced by:

- providing public information;
- possibly fencing off the upstream areas of the source and the collection point;
- use of water watchmen;
- keeping separate access points for watering animals.

Water treatment: If possible, avoid the need to treat water. If water is known to be polluted and chlorination is not possible, the quickest treatment is to pump water into open storage tanks and hold for as long as possible before distribution (six hours minimum). Water quality improves if water is stored and allowed to stand. For domestic use, leaving water in transparent containers in sunlight for four to five hours improves water quality, if the water is not too turbid.

Chlorination: When there is a fully operational water programme, it is best to keep all water chlorinated with a reasonable residual so that there is an effect on the water being collected and when the water is being stored in the household containers. Chlorine is a widely available substance and is relatively cheap, but chlorine is only effective if the water turbidity levels are relatively low (see Appendix 6). Chlorine levels can be measured with a simple pool tester. If large-scale water chlorination is considered, technical advice should be sought.

Hygiene promotion: Pollution often occurs at household level from dirty or uncovered storage vessels, or inappropriate handling of the water. Hygiene promotion is very important, to ensure that refugees understand the importance of hygienic practices, and that they have suitable, covered water containers for carrying and storing water. Lids for containers will reduce the chance of contamination.

Sanitation and waste disposal
The failure to dispose of faeces safely is a major cause of refugee ill-health and can lead to epidemics. Sanitation is a difficult part of the health programme and is often poorly implemented, or ignored. It is vital to involve refugees from the outset if sanitation interventions are to be effective. Women should be consulted and involved in planning the type and the location of facilities, and the sanitation programme should be co-ordinated closely with the health and water programme. Promotion of improved hygiene practices is integral to the sanitation programme.

Immediate action: If it is not too late, the initial camp layout should be planned to allow space for the construction of family or group latrines. Attempts to build latrines in already established camps are usually much less successful, but should still be a priority.

In the absence of any system, demarcated defecation areas should be identified to avoid indiscriminate defecation and possible pollution of water sources. The area should be at least 50 metres away from shelters, and if feasible, shovels provided for individual or group cleaning of the area.

Trench latrines may be considered but these are often unacceptable and poorly maintained.

Latrine construction: Pit latrines are usually the most appropriate option. Family latrines are more acceptable and better maintained than community latrines. The ratio should be one latrine for 20 people. Construction should be in phases to achieve this target, whilst ensuring equal coverage (first phase, one latrine for 200 people; second phase, one latrine for 100 people, and so on).

Latrines should be sited as far away as possible from the water source, particularly if this is a surface water source (pond or river). The minimum distance in sandy or loamy soil is 15 metres, more in shallow soil or rocky areas. Latrines should be down hill of water sources.

Consider the need for privacy and security, especially for women. Water should be made available for anal cleansing (where used) and for handwashing.

Latrine maintenance: Latrines need to be cleaned daily, and regularly maintained. Responsibilities for this should be assigned, in consultation with refugees. When full, latrines must be closed and alternative latrines opened. Where space is very limited, full latrines may be emptied by suction tanker.

Women's needs: Besides the need for privacy and security when using latrines, women's requirements for sanitary material for menstrual protection should be considered.

Children's needs: Arrangements should be made for toddlers and small children. Toddler latrines may be considered, and a hygiene campaign to clean up toddlers' faeces and safely dispose of them.

Disposal of solid waste: Safe disposal of waste is important, because insects and rats spread infection from contaminated organic material. Organise communal collection if possible, and encourage people to dig pits for family waste, and cover with earth.

Market places should be sited well away from shelters, and waste from markets collected, and buried or burnt.

Waste from health centres is particularly dangerous. It should be handled carefully and destroyed daily in an incinerator, and any residue buried in a pit.

Disposal of liquid waste: Provision for the disposal of liquid waste must be made, particularly from washing areas in camps. A simple soak pit for waste water should be constructed.

Vector control

There are numerous vector-borne diseases. Flies are transmitters of diarrhoea and trachoma, mechanically, but there are other ways of acquiring infection e.g. direct faecal contamination of food, rubbing eyes, or eating, with contaminated hands. In the case of other diseases, the vector is the only way in which a specific disease can be transmitted, as it is a necessary part of the life-cycle of the pathogen. Malaria, transmitted by *Anopheles* mosquitoes, is by far the most important vector-borne disease worldwide. Others of significance in some refugee contexts are: scabies (mites), dengue (mosquitoes), yellow fever (mosquitoes), typhus and relapsing fever (lice), sleeping sickness (tsetse fly) river blindness or onchocerciasis (black flies), leishmaniasis (sand flies). The snail which hosts schistosomiasis is not a vector in the strict sense, as infection occurs from free-swimming larvae of the fluke after they have left the snail.

Vector-borne diseases may be exacerbated in refugee populations because, unlike the local population, refugees may lack immunity to, for example, malaria. Refugees may have fled through an infested area (sleeping sickness, visceral leishmaniasis) or settled on land uninhabited by local population because of vector presence (river blindness). Refugees may live in unhygienic and crowded camps, where diarrhoeal diseases, trachoma, typhus, and scabies can spread rapidly; stress and malnutrition may exacerbate morbidity. In addition, particularly in situations of armed conflict, the national vector control programme may have broken down locally or nationally.

Before planning a specific vector control programme, it is important to gather information on which vectors are likely to occur in the local environment. Correct diagnosis of the disease and the vector is vital.

Water engineers must be aware of the need for environmental management around the water supplies they arrange. They should take responsibility for eliminating stagnant pools where mosquitoes can breed.

Important components of vector control are:
• choice of camp location;
• appropriate shelter;
• public awareness and education;
• maintenance of water supply system;
• adequate sanitation;
• environmental management: clearing scrub, drainage;
• personal hygiene;
• use of bednets;
• use of insect repellents;
• chemical control methods.

Periodically, campaigns against specific vectors may become necessary. Coordinated public information, mass mobilisation to eliminate vector breeding-grounds, and mass treatment can eliminate or drastically reduce the disease, at least temporarily.

Note that spraying is only one of a range of control methods. It is expensive, and is often only partial and temporary. If spraying is considered, the programme has to be planned in detail, in co-operation with the Ministry of Health and local health authorities, and discussed beforehand with the refugees. Equipment should be of good quality and the correct and safe insecticide and application method chosen.

Monitoring: The effectiveness of environmental health interventions can be monitored through indicators of health status in terms of incidence and prevalence of water and vector-related diseases, technical indicators such as water availability per capita, and latrine capacity, and indicators relating to hygiene behaviour at community, household or individual level, such as use of latrines, uptake of ORT, hand-washing practices.

Shelter

Inadequate and overcrowded shelter is a major factor in the transmission of communicable disease. The recommended (WHO) minimum usable floor space in an emergency is 3.5 square metres per person. The distance between shelters should at least be sufficient to prevent the spread of fire, and to allow for drainage. Latrines should be at least 6 metres from the living area, but no further than 50 metres.

In provision of shelter material the following requirements must be considered: designs and constructions with which the refugees are familiar; the availability of local materials and environmental consequences; cultural norms, and needs for privacy, washing and cooking areas. It is also important to consider the need for shelter against both rain and sun. In some places, rudimentary emergency shelters will need to be strengthened to protect refugees from severe winter conditions of sub-zero temperatures, snow, and ice.

Re-inforced plastic sheeting can be used for roofing and flooring. Blankets may be used as additional roofing, or as screening inside the shelter to afford more privacy.

2.3.2 Immunisation

An immunisation campaign against measles should be regarded as a priority in any large refugee programme, even if the population have fled from a country with high immunisation coverage.

During the initial emergency phase all children aged six months to five years should be vaccinated. Children vaccinated between six and nine months must be re-vaccinated after reaching nine months of age. In some situations, it may be necessary to vaccinate children up to 12 years of age. At other times the minimum age can be increased to nine months. The coverage rate should be at least 95 per cent to prevent an outbreak.

Undernutrition, fever, diarrhoea, respiratory infections are *not* contraindications to vaccination. Measles vaccine should also be given to people with HIV infection and active TB.

Vitamin A deficiency: This may increase mortality and is a particular risk in combination with measles and diarrhoea, which deplete bodily stores of vitamin A. Vitamin A deficiency also causes xerophthalmia which can lead to blindness.

Low reserves of vitamin A are so common among children in the first phase of a refugee emergency that routine vitamin A supplementation in conjunction with a measles immunisation campaign is recommended. This has the further practical advantage that administration can be recorded together with immunisation on the health card and in the central register. It is also necessary to establish a system to maintain coverage, involving screening of new arrivals to the camp and registration and follow-up of new births.

Meningitis: In areas where epidemics of meningococcal meningitis occur, emergency meningitis immunisation may become necessary.

Additional immunisations: Immunisation against other vaccine-preventable diseases is not an immediate emergency measure. However, it is recommended if the population is expected to remain stable for at least three months, if the operational capacity exists, and if it can be integrated in the national Expanded Programme for Immunisation (EPI) within a reasonable time. These services would be best delivered out of a mother-and-child-health (MCH) clinic. Apart from measles vaccine, the vaccines included in most EPI programmes are those against polio, diphtheria, pertussis, tetanus and tuberculosis (see Appendix 9 for details of doses, and schedules).

Cold chain: If an effective local immunisation programme exists in the host country, it should be possible either to use the local cold-chain facilities or to give some assistance to up-grade them. If there is no local immunisation programme or cold- chain facility, special arrangements to maintain the cold chain up to the site of the camp will have to be made.

Organising an immunisation campaign: Elements in the organisation and management of an immunisation campaign are:

- public information and mobilisation;
- assigning responsibility for different aspects of the campaign to refugee leaders and agencies;
- procurement of supplies;
- pre-registration of children, if possible;
- organising facilities for vaccine administration;
- administration of vaccines;
- recording and reporting, and evaluating.

Adequate immunisation records should be kept; these should include personal immunisation cards (e.g. 'Road to Health' cards) and a central register.

Monitoring: The effectiveness of an immunisation programme can be assessed from observation of the process and information in the central register, MCH returns, and population-based surveys.

2.3.3 Health promotion

Health promotion in the broadest sense encompasses social, political, and economic changes, in addition to behaviour change at community and individual level if that behaviour is causing ill health.

A health promotion programme which focuses on hygiene promotion at community, household and personal level, is an important and integral part of a refugee health programme, and not an optional extra. Refugees may find themselves in a situation with greatly increased risks to their health, to which they have not yet developed adequate responses. For example, in their own environment, defecation in the fields or in wasteland surrounding their homes may be perfectly safe, whereas in a crowded camp environment the same practice would represent a serious health hazard. Natural water sources may become rapidly contaminated through over-use. Crowding may lead to an increased incidence in communicable diseases. Social dislocation and rape may have led to an increase in STDs, including HIV/AIDS.

Content of a health promotion programme: This will be determined by the specific health risk factors in the new environment. The cultural background and practices of the population must be taken into account. It is important that the programme is adapted to cover new health problems as they arise.

Methods of health promotion: There are many ways in which health promotion is carried out: health education to individuals attending clinics, to groups gathered together specially for the purpose, and by public information through posters and announcements. The use of drama, and songs can be very effective. In addition, public action and lobbying to campaign for better facilities might be considered. Health education messages should be kept simple and methods must be culturally appropriate and non-judgmental. It is particularly important that women have access to health information and that the messages and methods of the programme do not imply blame for their own or their children's ill health.

2.4 Control of communicable diseases

In the long term, the control of communicable diseases depends on a healthy environment (clean water, adequate sanitation, vector control, adequate shelter: see section 2.3.1 Environmental health), immunisation, and the training of health workers in early diagnosis and treatment (see section 2.7 Training). In principle, the three main methods of control are dealing with the source of infection; interrupting transmission; and protecting susceptible individuals:

2.4.1 Summary of main methods for controlling diseases

1 Attacking source of infection by:

    treatment of cases and carriers

    isolation of cases

    surveillance of suspected cases

    notification of cases to authorities

    control of animal reservoirs of disease

2 Interrupting transmission by:

    environmental health action: water supplies, excreta disposal, food hygiene, vector control, personal hygiene

    disinfection and sterilisation of surroundings

    reduction of crowding, population movements and migration

3 Protecting susceptible individuals by:

    immunisation

    chemo-prophylaxis

    personal protection

    improved nutrition

2.4.2 Investigating disease outbreaks (epidemics)

An epidemic is an unusually large or unexpected increase in the number of cases of a disease for a given place and time period. An epidemiological investigation should be conducted to confirm the existence of an epidemic, and identify the causative agent, its source, and mode of transmission.

Many infectious diseases require laboratory facilities for adequate diagnosis and for the collection of epidemiological data. A simple camp laboratory with microscopy will be an asset, but many outbreak investigations require more sophisticated equipment and skills. These will usually be available only at regional, national, or even international level. But even so, camp laboratory technicians will play an important role in collecting, storing, and dispatching specimens. Suitable sterile containers and transport media should be pre-positioned at the camp laboratory. Data collected on the number of cases, and characteristics of the people affected, should be analysed to identify those most at risk. With this data and an assessment of local response capacity, the most effective control measures possible should be implemented. It is essential to keep the community informed of findings and plans for control.

The specific control measures taken will depend on the type of epidemic. Emergency treatment centres may be required for cholera or dysentery, for example, which will require extra resources. If poorly managed, such centres will have little impact on case-fatality rates and may deter cases from presenting.

2.4.3 Control of common diseases

Communicable diseases which are also the commonest causes of excess mortality and morbidity among refugees are measles; diarrhoeal diseases, including watery diarrhoea, cholera, and bacillary dysentery; acute lower respiratory tract infections (ALRIs); and malaria. Other communicable diseases which have caused special concern in refugee settings in recent years include meningococcal meningitis, scabies, hepatitis, trachoma, typhoid, and typhus, TB and HIV/AIDS.

Measles
Every individual who has not either had the disease or been immunised is susceptible. The only effective control measure for measles is immunisation.

In the case of a measles outbreak immunisation should be accelerated, because people who have been exposed to infection may be partially protected if the vaccine is administered within three days.

There is no effective treatment for measles, and isolation of cases has no effect on the spread of the disease. For managing individual cases, the main actions are to treat complications (which might include diarrhoea, acute respiratory infections, and otitis) and give nutritional supplements and vitamin A. WHO now recommend that children with 'complicated measles' receive two consecutive doses of vitamin A.

Diarrhoeal diseases
The main control measures are the provision of a clean water supply, effective sanitation and hygiene education. A clear case-definition of diarrhoea should be established e.g. at least three loose or watery stools in one day.

Acute watery diarrhoea: Many different organisms can cause watery diarrhoea, and patients usually recover spontaneously as long as dehydration is prevented. It is dehydration which causes diarrhoea-related deaths. Oral rehydration is the effective treatment in the vast majority of patients, including those suffering from cholera (Appendix 8). It is also important to maintain nutrition.

Cholera: Profuse watery diarrhoea often with vomiting, affecting all age groups. It can spread very quickly and result in severe dehydration within hours of onset. It is therefore important to be prepared and have already pre-positioned:

• extra supplies of ORS, IV fluids and appropriate antibiotics;
• health workers trained in management of cholera.

If the attack (incidence) rate is high the following measures will be required:
- establishing temporary cholera-wards to cope with the patient load;
- active case finding;
- daily reporting of new cases and deaths (including location in camp, and length of stay in camp);
- intensive health education and public information campaign.

Mass chemoprophylaxis is **not** recommended as a control measure. If resources are adequate and transmission rates high, a single dose of doxycycline may be given to members of the immediate family of cases.

Dysentery: Diarrhoea with visible blood in the stool. The two major types are caused by amoeba and shigella. The latter (shigellosis) represents the greater health risk. It is endemic in many poor communities, and can occur in epidemic outbreaks, especially in conditions of overcrowding and bad sanitation. Prompt treatment with antibiotics is a control measure as it decreases the severity, and duration of excretion of the pathogen. However, treatment may be complicated by resistant strains of shigella, so the choice of drug must be based on local susceptibility patterns (Appendix 8).

Mass chemoprophylaxis or chemoprophylaxis of family members is **not** recommended as a control measure for shigellosis.

Malaria

Worldwide, malaria is by far the most important of all vector-borne diseases. Refugees are often particularly vulnerable.

Vector control, including elimination of breeding sites, use of insecticides, and personal protection, including the use of bed-nets, is the principal component of a malaria control programme. Prompt and effective treatment of malaria reduces the parasite reservoir (see Appendix 8 for treatment guidelines for fever). Although fever in the absence of other focal signs and symptoms is usually treated as malaria in areas and seasons of high transmission, this does mean that a large number of patients are treated for malaria whose fever is due to other causes. Proper diagnosis is by microscopic blood film examination, which should be available in camp laboratories wherever transmission occurs.

Chloroquine is still effective in many parts of Africa. However, where the malaria parasite has developed resistance, alternative drugs, such as mefloquine, must be used. Recommended choice of drugs and regimens vary and should be ascertained locally (see Appendix 8).

Chemoprophylaxis protects against disease, not against infection. If the refugee health care system has the capacity, and if at-risk persons can be readily identified, chemoprophylaxis may be considered. Groups at particular risk from the

34

complications of malaria are children under five, especially the malnourished and sick, pregnant women, and other groups with poor health status.

Acute lower respiratory infection (ALRI)

Acute infections of the lower respiratory tract are a major cause of child mortality in poor countries. A large proportion of these infections are bacterial, so prompt treatment with an appropriate antibiotic will reduce mortality. ALRI is a common complication of measles, and also a consequence of crowding and inadequate shelter. Distribution of blankets and children's clothing will help to reduce susceptibility. Health education in clinics and at household level on the management of fever and dehydration is an important element in reducing mortality.

It is essential that health workers agree and follow clear case-definitions and have clear criteria, treatment, and referral protocols for moderate and severe cases. The main sign of the presence of pneumonia in children is a respiration rate of more than 50 per minute, and the main sign of severity is chest indrawing.

Hepatitis

In refugee camps, outbreaks of acute viral hepatitis A may occur. Prevention and control measures are improvements in water and sanitation provision and personal hygiene, as transmission is faecal-oral. The most common sign in cases is jaundice. There is no treatment, though local treatments may offer symptomatic relief.

Meningococcal meningitis

Meningitis is endemic in most of the world. Periodic epidemics occur, particularly in what is known as the 'meningitis belt' across sub-Saharan Africa north of the equator, at intervals of 8 to 12 years, although the intervals have shortened in several countries, and in recent years the disease has also spread into East Africa. The epidemics tend to break out at the end of the dry season and end soon after the beginning of the rains.

It is difficult to define the threshold of an outbreak, because endemic rates vary by geographic area, season, and patient characteristics. One suggestion for a rough indicator of a meningitis outbreak is a doubling of the baseline number of cases from one week to the next over a period of three weeks.

Surveillance is the key to control of the disease. For effective surveillance, a standard case definition must be applied by all health workers. There should also be a clearly established reporting network.

Diagnosis is by bacteriological examination of cerebro-spinal fluid (CSF). This also establishes the serotype and sensitivity of the organism. After an outbreak has been confirmed, a presumptive diagnosis in people with suggestive signs and symptoms (severe headache, vomiting, photophobia, fever, neck stiffness), can be made from visual inspection of CSF.

Once an outbreak has been identified, an immunisation campaign should be started, first focusing on the area and families where cases have occurred. Vaccines exist for serotype A and C, and all epidemics in Africa have been caused by one or other of these. Immunisation during non-epidemic periods is not recommended, except if there is reason to believe that the refugees are at high risk for an epidemic. No form of chemoprophylaxis is recommended against epidemic meningitis.

Treatment in refugee settings where intensive nursing care is not available, is by a single intra-muscular injection of chloramphenicol. However, patients should be closely monitored, because in 25 per cent of patients a second injection is needed.

Tuberculosis
Off all single pathogens the TB bacillus is responsible for most deaths worldwide. WHO estimates 8 to 10 million new cases and 3 million deaths per year. The vast majority of these are in the countries of the South. Transmission is increased by poor housing and poverty, making refugees particularly vulnerable

Although most tuberculosis is curable, the difficulty lies in establishing a well-organised programme in which patients complete the prolonged treatment. The instability of many refugee camps makes this even more difficult than it is in other settings with poor health services, and an ambitious active case-finding programme is unlikely to be successful. If the decision to commence a TB programme is made, then a policy should be agreed by all organisations providing health services, covering case definition, case-finding, treatment regimen, and supervision of chemotherapy.

Transmission is through sputum-positive patients. 'Sputum-positive' means patients whose sputum shows acid-fast bacilli (AFB) on microscopy of specimens stained by the Ziehl-Neelsen method. Efforts should concentrate on control of transmission through treatment of these patients.

Passive-casefinding, i.e. testing the sputum of people presenting at health facilities with suggestive symptoms (cough of more than three weeks' duration, chest pain, haemoptysis, weight loss) is the most appropriate. Symptomatic family contacts of confirmed cases should also be sputum-tested. Symptomatic children may not be sputum-positive although they suffer from the disease. They should be given a full course of treatment, if they are close contacts of a confirmed TB patient, or a tuberculin skin test is strongly positive, in the absence of a BCG scar.

If possible, the treatment regimen should be consistent with the national policy in the host country. However, because high rates of transmission are likely and because the duration of stay of the refugees is uncertain, short-course therapy (six months) should be considered, even if the national policy prescribes a longer course of treatment (up to 18 months). In addition, short-course therapy includes rifampicin, and avoids the need for streptomycin, which has to be administered by injection. Other drugs used are isoniazid, pyrazinamide, ethambutol and thiacetazone. Depending on local conditions, three or four drugs will be used in combination. Specific therapeutic regimens will have to be agreed locally, with UNHCR, other agencies, and MoH.

Case-holding is an important part of tuberculosis control, as incomplete treatment encourages the emergence of drug-resistant strains. Pre-requisites for successful case-holding are:

- supervised treatment, especially during the first two to three months;
- record system;
- defaulter tracing;
- clear assignment of responsibilities;
- public information and health promotion.

BCG vaccination plays an important role in protecting children from TB meningitis and miliary TB. The degree of protection afforded against pulmonary TB is disputed. Vaccination with BCG should therefore be part of the comprehensive immunisation programme, not a separate TB-control activity. BCG is contraindicated for persons with symptomatic HIV infection.

HIV/AIDS
Disruption and migration have been linked to increased transmission of HIV, but there is so far no evidence that HIV and AIDS affect refugees more than other groups. The rate of infection is likely to be similar to that among the community before displacement. It is important to avoid labelling an already marginalised group who can easily become a target for suspicion and hostility. It is important that refugees are included in the HIV/AIDS programme of the host country, or that the issue is addressed by refugee health services. Health promotion round HIV/AIDS issues should be integrated with other health promotion activities.

In some countries, legal and human rights issues have become important in connection with AIDS. People with HIV or AIDS may be compulsorily screened; the exclusion from immigration programmes, or expulsion, is a growing problem. Agencies may have to become involved with issues surrounding the care, support and protection of refugees with AIDS.

Public information and health promotion, and making condoms widely available, are the principal means of prevention. Health education messages already developed in the host country or country of origin can be used. The training of traditional practitioners and community health workers is important, and also the protection of women refugees, especially if they are vulnerable to rape. The early diagnosis and adequate treatment of sexually transmitted diseases (STDs) is an important preventive measure, as there is a link between genital ulceration and HIV infection.

Care of patients should include good nutrition and the early diagnosis and treatment of infections. In countries with a high TB prevalence, HIV infection is often first identified when patients present with symptoms of TB. The confidentiality of patients should be respected, and relatives trained to care for the patient

2.5 Clinical care

2.5.1 Physical facilities, organisational structures, staffing
Clinical services in the refugee camps themselves usually do not go beyond primary level unless the camp or group of camps is very large and the necessary resources are available. Problems beyond the capacity of the local services are referred to the appropriate nearest secondary facility, which has been identified during the original assessment.

Health care should be delivered through a hierarchy of structures and services which mirror as far as possible the structures in the host country, or, if more appropriate, those in the refugees' home country. At camp level, each full-time community health worker commonly covers a population of up to 1,000 people, through home visits and working out of a small health post. The next level up might be the health centre or dispensary with catchment population up to 10,000.

The health centre at the camp will be the focal point for all health-related staff at the camp — preventive, clinical, administrative. If possible, health centres should provide the following facilities:

- waiting area: shaded, and with easy access;
- consultation space: providing privacy, writing space, basic hygiene, space for examination of patients, with separate arrangements for men and women;
- mother-and-child-health space: this could include main treatment facilities for women (see section 2.5.2 Health care for women and children);
- treatment room for small injuries, injections, etc: providing privacy, safe disposal of rubbish, equipment for injections;
- space for treatment of conditions with public health significance e.g. rehydration area;

- space or room for health education;
- small laboratory: for a limited range of basic tests;
- pharmacy: for dispensing of drugs;
- store for equipment and drugs: secure, and at the correct temperatures for drugs, with systematic stock taking;
- space for records and administration: standardised system through each level of referral.

Organisation of health centre

Patient flow: In the early days of an emergency clinical facilities are often overwhelmed by large numbers of patients. It is important that patient flow is properly organised to make the best use of staff time and facilities and avoid long waiting times. A system of triage may be required.

Screening patients is essential. Community health workers (CHWs) can deal with those presenting with trivial or simple complaints and refer other patients to the medical assistant or doctor. CHWs must have clear guidelines on whom to refer.

Access for women: If necessary, separate facilities for women may be required or arranging different times for men and women to attend clinics. Women find it especially difficult to consult about gynaecological problems or STDs and every effort must be made to provide privacy. In some cultures it is essential to provide female health staff.

Supply system: a regular supply of consumable items, such as cotton wool, bandages, disinfectants, soap and drugs, must be arranged. Arrangements for the maintenance of equipment, including a supply of spare parts, are essential for the functioning of the health service.

Systems for managing stores, and stock keeping must be set up.

Referral facilities: local health services, perhaps already overstretched, understaffed and inadequately equipped, often cannot cope with the additional work due to refugees being referred for treatment which cannot be provided in the camp. If this is the case, local health services should be strengthened, by, for example, providing additional personnel or incentives for extra work, increased drug supplies, and food for patient meals. This could also help to improve relations with the local population, probably very poor themselves, who are likely to feel resentful if the refugees are seen to enjoy better facilities than they do. A similar problem occurs if refugees receive free health care whilst locals pay a fee. Large hospitals should not be set up in camps. However a small in-patient facility (5-10 beds) may be required to give emergency treatment pending the patient's referral to a hospital or return home.

Staffing

The largest item on the budget of a health service is usually staff salaries. Every effort should be made to identify suitable and skilled workers from the refugee population itself, as they are familiar with the culture and language of the group. Special consideration should also be given to women in the recruitment and training of health workers, because women and children form the majority in most refugee populations, and women health workers have better access to other women. Training can empower women, through the acquisition of skills, and consequent earning capacity, and participation in community work. Categories of health workers are given below.

Community-based:
1 Helpers and ancillary workers in sanitation and waste disposal, feeding programmes, food stores. They will usually be refugees, and need only minimal training. They need the visible support and backing of the health professionals, to increase the effectiveness of their work.
2 Traditional birth attendants (TBAs), trained and supervised at MCH centre.
3 Community health workers (CHWs), covering between 100 and 1000 of the population (the ratio depends on a number of variables such as resources available, geographical distribution, expectations and past experience of refugees).
4 Traditional healers from the refugee community, who may be, for example, herbalists, bone-setters, holy men and women, or shamans. They offer services for cash or payment in kind.
5 There may also be pharmacists and drug retailers within the refugee population who operate on a commercial basis.

Clinic-based:
1 Midwife at Mother-and-child Health Centre (plus TBAs).
2 Trained nurses and nursing auxiliaries/dressers (plus CHWs).
3 Laboratory technicians, pharmacist, nutritionist.
4 Medical assistant or physician.

Health coordinator: This may be the medical assistant or physician, if s/he has relevant professional experience. There may be a hierarchy of co-ordinators from camp level to district to national level. A logistics capacity, for transport of people and supplies, is also required at each level.

Monitoring

The effectiveness of clinical care can be monitored through clinic returns, morbidity surveillance, and records of drug consumption. Periodic surveys to assess uptake may be necessary.

2.5.2 Health care for women and children

Women's health care should include:-

- screening for high risk pregnancy (provided referral facilities are available);
- immunisation against tetanus;
- iron and folic acid supplementation during pregnancy, as well as iodine in areas of endemic goitre;
- screening for anaemia;
- birth planning;
- treatment of sexually transmitted disease (STDs);
- counselling for victims of violence, especially rape;
- preventive and curative services, including gynaecological care;
- health education both about their own health and that of their children.

It is important that provision is made for obstetric emergencies. Pregnancy and birth are risky even in normal circumstances in poor communities: it is estimated that, globally, 500,000 women die in childbirth every year. Many refugee women are malnourished and may have suffered violence or mental trauma in the recent past, all of which may increase the risk in pregnancy. At a minimum, the nearest surgical facility should be identified and if possible, standby transport arranged.

These services, or some of them, are usually provided jointly with health care for children in the form of mother-and-child-health (MCH) services. However, MCH services focus on pregnant women and children under five years of age and so exclude women who are not pregnant or who are childless. Wherever possible, MCH should be broadened to include health care for all women.

There should be one MCH clinic per approximately 5000 population, to provide routine screening, preventive, and curative services to women and to children under two years of age. The age range is sometimes extended to include all children under five years old. The MCH centre should liaise with other services and social networks for women and children outside the health sector.

Services for children include:

- screening for e.g. scabies, anaemia;
- nutritional assessment;
- nutritional rehabilitation and food supplementation;
- immunisation and vitamin A supplementation;
- rehydration for children suffering from diarrhoea;
- curative care.

MCH centres should be staffed by trained female personnel. In most cases the staff will include a nurse-midwife, who can also support and supervise traditional birth attendants (TBAs). TBAs should be identified among the refugees, trained and given supplies. Their major tasks are the recognition of women with high-risk pregnancies, carrying out safe, hygienic delivery, and follow-up of mothers and babies at home. They should be trained to report perinatal mortality.

Monitoring
This can be done through clinic returns, attendance registers, immunisation registers, maternal mortality rates, and under-five mortality rates.

2.5.3 Laboratory facilities
A simple camp laboratory fulfils a double role; firstly, as mentioned in section 2.4.2, in disease surveillance and outbreak investigations; and secondly, as an essential tool for rational clinical care.

A laboratory technician will be needed, and the most important piece of equipment is a standard light microscope. A relatively small range of tests covers most important clinical needs and will usually include microscopy of:
* stools — amoeba, giardia, worms;
* urine — urinary tract infections;
* blood — malaria, white cell count, blood film appearance;
* sputum — Ziehl-Neelsen for acid-fast bacilli (tuberculosis);
* pus and smears — gram stain;
* cerebro-spinal fluid (if lumbar puncture can be done) — meningitis organisms.

The selection of tests will vary according to local conditions and morbidity profile.

A haemoglobinometer for haemoglobin estimation and supplies of dipsticks for urinary protein and glucose are especially useful for maternal care.

2.5.4 Essential drugs and equipment
Medicines and basic equipment are an expensive component of a refugee health programme, and often have to be bought with scarce hard currency. It is wasteful if inappropriate drugs and equipment are procured. Prescription practices must follow standard guidelines.

All programmes should have a commitment to an essential drug list, standard treatment guidelines, and rational prescribing. All prescribers should understand the basic principles involved. If this is not the case, training sessions for all health workers whose work includes prescribing should be organised as a priority. Untrained and unauthorised persons should not have access to the pharmacy or drug store.

Patient expectations often put pressure on prescribers to use drugs inappropriately. Health education and public information programmes should cover basic principles of the use and misuse of medicinal drugs and discourage the common irrational faith in injections.

Drug procurement

Drugs should only be procured from reputable sources; counterfeit and sub-standard drugs are an increasing problem on national and international markets. Unsolicited donations of drugs and equipment should not be accepted. They are often inappropriate for the needs of the programme, inadequately labelled, or nearing their expiry date.

Efficient systems for the management of drugs saves money and ensures that medicines are in a fit condition for people to use. Drug management includes appropriate transport and storage, systematic stocktaking and re-ordering, and ensuring security. Ensure there is a drug-use monitoring system that links morbidity-surveillance data with standard treatment-regimens.

WHO and other agencies have devised an 'Emergency Health Kit', which consists of drugs and equipment calculated for the needs of 10,000 people for three months. It is divided into two units, the 'Basic Unit', containing drugs and equipment in ten sub-units to be used by primary health care workers, each serving 1000 people; and the 'Supplementary Unit', to be used by professional health workers or physicians. A booklet, *The New Emergency Health Kit* (see Bibliography), contains a full contents list by generic names, with quantities, rationale for selection, as well as treatment guidelines and more detailed treatment plans for diarrhoea and acute respiratory infections (see Appendix 7 for summary of contents, Appendix 8 for treatment plans).

2.6 Psycho-social issues

The psycho-social effects of forced migration and displacement must be considered in the assessment, planning and implementation of health care. In the past they have often been ignored by health workers. However, there is a danger of 'medicalising' psychological and social reactions to extreme and horrific experiences. Distress is a normal consequence of having experienced violent incidents, protracted harassment, or having been forced to leave one's home because of drought and famine.

How people react to this kind of stress is shaped by cultural norms and expectations. The health worker should focus on the individual's ability to function and survive in the new context, not on psychological signs and symptoms.

2.6.1 Identification of vulnerable groups

Individuals and groups who may be particularly distressed and unable to function socially are likely to be known to the community. They may include:

- people whose relatives have been killed or are missing;
- children who have been exposed to violence to themselves or witnessed atrocities being perpetrated on members of their family;
- people who have been subjected to systematic torture, including rape;
- women alone with small children, vulnerable to sexual violence during their flight and in the camp itself;
- men who have been repeatedly exposed to combat and involved in committing atrocities;
- people physically disabled by violence.

2.6.2 Rehabilitation

An important factor in rehabilitation and prevention of severe long-term disorder is social cohesion. The health worker can promote this through participating in the refugee community life, structures and social groups, working together with the camp administration, local host government officers and other agencies to try and ensure that the camp provides a secure, safe environment, free from harassment.

Refugee involvement in planning and implementation of programmes, including participation of women, is important, as it helps to promote some level of autonomy and control over their situation.

Services must be readily accessible for all groups, especially for those who may need extra support to function socially such as the disabled, unaccompanied children, widowed women, and marginalised minorities.

Strengthening community coping mechanisms

Existing social networks and traditional coping mechanisms, religious rituals, burial rites, and other expressions of cultural identity, should be recognised and fostered. Practical measures might include the following:-

- provision of play areas and schooling for children;
- provision of traditional burial cloth;
- ensuring meeting rooms are available;
- repair of churches and care for holy places;
- organising tracing of missing family members, especially for orphans;
- provision of prostheses and aids for disabled.

Listening to the testimony of people about human rights abuses, and where possible and safe, documenting the effects and human costs of war can be valuable, and may lead to advocacy, where appropriate.

2.6.3 Training in awareness of psychosocial issues

The training of health workers should include awareness raising and discussion on how to support those people who are so distressed that they can no longer function as before in their role for example as parents or community leaders. Such people may present at the health post. Health worker training should therefore emphasise the importance of a respectful approach and sensitivity to the patient's own belief systems, and the need to protect the patient from being stigmatised or labelled.

Networks and social support systems are very important, and health facilities such as MCH or supplementary feeding centres may provide the opportunity and setting for women in particular to meet and find support from each other.

Health workers should understand that some mild physical conditions, such as headache, general body pain, fatigue, episodic breathing difficulties, might be psycho-somatic presentations, and try to avoid giving medication which is not needed. They also need to know how and when to refer patients elsewhere, such as to wise elders, religious leaders, traditional healers, or for drug therapy, and how to provide humane and appropriate care for the mentally ill.

2.6.4 Post-traumatic stress disorder (PTSD)
Post-traumatic stress disorder (PTSD) is a classification of mental disorder in individuals who have suffered a traumatic experience. Symptoms include sleep disturbance, mood lability, fatigue, and hypervigilance. Symptoms may not appear for several months after the event and may persist for years. However, these symptoms may or may not affect the individual's ability to function socially.

PTSD belongs to a Western model of psychiatric classification. Symptoms which are considered to be part of the disorder may have different meanings for people from other cultures and, conversely, people form other cultures may not exhibit these symptoms. For example, sleep disturbance may have a healing effect for people for whom dreams and nightmares are links with ancestors and kind spirits.

2.6.5 Monitoring
Monitoring of an individual's improved ability to function will be through observation and their personal history. Monitoring how much the refugees collectively are recovering could be done through a variety of methods from observation, discussion, and study of individual case histories, to looking at proxy quantitative indicators such as economic and social activity.

2.7 Training

There are usually some trained health workers among the refugees. They should be identified and recruited if appropriate. It may, however, be necessary to provide additional training to equip these health workers for work in the refugee situation, or to train newly-recruited workers. Special consideration should be given to the recruitment and training of women.

2.7.1 Training needs
Training needs will vary depending largely on the type of health worker, the status of their previous training, and how recently they received training. Trained professionals, usually doctors and nurses, will have been trained in formal hospital settings. They may now require additional training and re-orientation in preventive aspects of health care, and rational prescribing.

Community-based health workers may require new or refresher training, which should be based on clear job descriptions, and close supervision and support 'on the job' should be integral to their training programme. Formal training may be inappropriate for traditional healers, but workshops and meetings can be arranged to share information, discuss possible cross-referral mechanisms, and to build mutual trust;

Auxiliary staff will require specific and minimal training to perform tasks, for example, in feeding centres, or in the maintenance of water-supply systems, or camp cleaning.

.2.7.2 Training issues
Before beginning a training programme, clarity and agreement must be reached between camp authorities, trainers and trainees about some questions which frequently become contentious:
- Are job descriptions available, including task analysis?
- Will the health workers be paid or work on a voluntary basis?
- Is the programme sustainable? (Especially important if salaries are involved.)
- How will the trainees be selected and recruited and who will recruit them?
- How long will the training programme last and what training methods will be used, what will the content be, and what materials will be required?
- How will the health workers be supervised and supported, and who by?

2.7.3 Training methods
The training programme must be framed around learning objectives which arise from the health workers' job descriptions. In most situations, primary health workers' tasks will include the following:
- collection of birth and mortality data;
- food and feeding programmes, including identification of malnutrition;
- immunisations;
- practical steps to improve environmental health;

- prevention and treatment of diarrhoea;
- prevention and treatment of scabies;
- active case-finding for specific disease-control programmes;
- prevention and treatment of malaria;
- recognition of acute respiratory diseases;
- first aid;
- identification, support and referral of sick, isolated, disabled people;
- the rational use of essential drugs.

Training usually involves a range of methods, including some didactic teaching, participatory learning, role play, and supervised practice. Trainers among the refugee population should be involved in training activities. The training of trainers should be a major programme component.

3 Issues arising from long-term displacement

3.1 Introduction

When the acute phase passes and the situation of the refugees becomes 'chronic', a different set of problems will develop. Frequently, funds become less easily available as media interest wanes and aid organisations scale down operations, directing their attention to new emergencies elsewhere. There may be a move to reduce the level of aid, although the majority of the refugees are still dependent on relief. Any scaling down of relief operations must be done in a planned way, with government agencies, multilaterals and NGOs cooperating to develop clear criteria aimed at retaining vital services for those who do stay.

Fears in the host country that the refugees will stay forever may lead to pressure for repatriation and develop into a difficult political issue, influenced by many considerations beyond the control of the refugees and NGOs. For the purposes of this chapter we shall assume basic security and stability.

Greater stability may, of course, bring benefits for the welfare of the refugees. A proportion of the refugees may leave the camp, either to return home, to settle and find jobs locally, or disperse to live with relatives, decreasing crowding in the camp. Land in the area of the camp may be allocated for agriculture and gardening, giving opportunities for diversifying the food basket.

On the other hand, small numbers of refugees often continue to arrive in the camp for many months after the events which initiated the original influx. It is important, therefore, that a screening mechanism continues to exist which assesses the health status of newcomers. In some situations, for example when the camps have reached their planned capacity, late arrivals are not officially allowed to stay, and are perhaps denied ration cards and other official papers. They may thus try to avoid health screening for fear of exposure. Health workers must be on the lookout for groups of such people, who are particularly vulnerable.

With time, refugee and displaced camps often take on the character of an urban slum. Temporary shelters and emergency water supply and sanitation, which were adequate for the original emergency situation, deteriorate and will have to be replaced by some more permanent structures, if they are not to develop into health hazards. The ecological impact on the locality may be severe: there may be soil erosion, and stagnant water and accumulating rubbish may lead to an increase in vector-borne diseases. Deforestation due to fuel gathering in the camp vicinity will have direct implications for women who will have to walk further and further from the camp, increasing their work burden and facing an added security risk, from landmines, extortion, and violence, including rape.

3.2 Health Information Systems

Where possible, the Health Information System should be integrated into a national system, while retaining the capacity to pick up new trends which may emerge as the morbidity profile shifts over time. The system must remain sensitive to this. Long-term, the HIS will rely more on routinely collected information than on frequent, population-based surveys. This assumes an efficient record-keeping and monitoring system at health and feeding centres. The health workers must be motivated and trained to understand the significance of the paperwork they are asked to undertake, and the health authorities must analyse the information and feed it back to the health workers in usable form.

3.3 Nutrition

It will remain crucial to monitor nutritional status. However, it should become possible to lengthen the interval between population-based surveys, making more extensive use of nutrition data from MCH centres. However, growth-monitoring data from clinics is more likely to be biased as it only includes those children who regularly attend the MCH clinic, and excludes those for whom access is difficult. Also, growth monitoring data may not be directly comparable with the results of nutritional surveys because a different nutritional index is used. Growth monitoring uses the weight-for-age index, which reflects both wasting (acute malnutrition) and stunting (chronic malnutrition), while most surveys use the weight-for-height nutritional index which reflects wasting. While nutrition status remains precarious, population-based weight-for-height surveys should be carried out at least once a year. A system of monitoring the take-home ration should be established, for example, checking a random sample of 50 families each distribution day.

3.3.1 Food rations

General food rations tend to fluctuate in quantity, and delivery may be irregular. They may in any case be deficient in essential nutrients, with grave consequences for those refugees without the means to supplement the food baskets by earning cash incomes, bartering, or growing vegetables round their shelters. The onset of widespread micronutrient deficiencies is often insidious. The commonest are vitamin A deficiency and iron-deficiency anaemia, both of which are major public health problems in many poor communities in normal circumstances. Deficiency diseases which in recent years have been associated particularly with refugee settings are vitamin C deficiency (scurvy) and thiamine deficiency (beri-beri). (See Appendix 4.)

3.3.2 Supplementary feeding programmes

Depending on local conditions, clear criteria and systems must be developed for scaling down and eventual closing down of supplementary feeding centres, for example:

- geographic coverage: if the refugees are dispersed in a number of camps over a wide area, centres are 'thinned out' rather than closing all centres in one area, so that access for the remaining malnourished children in the whole area is maintained;
- a minimum number of recipients below which the centre will close should be agreed on: the remaining children should then be transferred to MCH centres for individual follow-up;
- the last centres to close should be those which serve newcomers.

3.4 Environmental health

Priorities will shift from emergency water and sanitation measures to issues of appropriate technology, maintenance and management.

The emergency water supply, which had to cope with the immediate need of large numbers, may be expensive, management-intensive and highly dependent on external inputs. In the long term, it will be necessary to find ways of supplying water which are more durable, controlled by users, and less expensive. For example, handpumps might be installed, especially if numbers in the camp decrease, and sand filtration, rather than flocculation and chlorination, used for water purification, because it needs less maintenance, does not need any chemicals, and uses local materials.

3.5 Immunisation

Immunisation among the refugee population should be subsumed into the local EPI programme, with the same attention to maintaining targets for coverage, as for normal programmes. Measles can be given at nine months of age, except during epidemics. The aim should be a 'supermarket' approach — where all services are available under one roof every day, so that opportunities for immunisation are not missed.

3.6 Health promotion

While health promotion in the acute phase may consist of a series of campaigns to reduce specific public health risks (e.g. scabies campaigns), perhaps with specialised campaign staff and volunteers, the emphasis will shift in the longer term to integrating health promotion into the health system, and towards using media closer to the culture of the refugees. The topics addressed will also change with time. Tuberculosis, alcohol and drug abuse, unemployment, child development in a camp environment, may replace the problems of the immediate emergency phase.

3.7 Disease control

The HIS must be sensitive enough to pick up new trends. Some communicable diseases, such as measles and malaria, are subject to seasonal changes and some, such as meningitis, can have a cyclical pattern extending over more than one year. The value of anecdotal reports should not be under-estimated. Delayed analysis of data is a common problem. New disease outbreaks may need to be investigated as they arise (see 2.4.2 Investigating disease outbreaks).

3.8 Disability

Disability may be a serious problem among refugees. In recent years, indiscriminate scattering of land mines in areas of conflict has caused enormous loss of life, and serious injury to hundreds of thousands of men, women and children. The possibility of death and disablement from land mines now represents a public health problem of great importance for returning refugee populations in many countries. With the breakdown of immunisation among the refugees, the incidence of poliomyelitis may have increased. Similarly, birth trauma due to difficult and unassisted births may have resulted in a greater number of children affected by cerebral palsy. The provision of physiotherapy and mobility aids, as well as skills training, will improve the quality of life for many refugees.

3.9 Clinical care

The potentially serious problem with clinical care in the long term is sustainability. The likely long-term solution will be integration into the host country structures. Meanwhile, capacity building through training of health staff among the refugees should be a priority. The Ministry of Health in the host country may need extra resources at central and district level to increase capacity. If the refugees begin to have some disposable income, it may be possible to safeguard drug supplies through a revolving drug fund or other community health-financing scheme.

3.10 Psycho-social issues

Problems such as alcoholism and drug abuse are likely to increase, especially for men deprived of status as breadwinners and protectors. There may be pressure to adapt to local customs in the host community, with a consequent loss of cultural identity; for example, women who have worn their traditional clothes may begin to feel ashamed of them and change their style of dress. Women may also have to adopt new roles to survive financially, and this may conflict with social and cultural norms. Children growing up with perhaps only dim memories of the old culture and way of life at home may become alienated from the older generation. The memory of trauma and violence, the lack of employment opportunities, and limited education facilities, may make the camps fertile recruiting grounds for armed factions and organised racketeering. Women may have had to resort to casual prostitution to earn cash. They may use the health-care network as an entry point for discussing their situation and other possible options.

With all the obvious disadvantages, it should also be remembered that the community life in a refugee camp may present opportunities for women to socialise and learn new skills, and for the education of children.

3.11 Training

Training of health workers will also have to adapt to long-term needs. Training for trainers will probably become more important, and NGOs may fund posts in appropriate Ministries in the host country to build long-term capacity. Proposals will probably be received by donors to fund key personnel secondments for training courses abroad.

At the other end of the scale, one of the greatest needs may be literacy teaching for women. Although this is not directly connected with the health programme, it has been shown that literacy and educational level is a significant variable for women's and children's health. Literacy training is most effective as part of a basic education programme and when linked to other opportunities, for example income generation where numeracy and literacy are important skills. Literacy classes have been used as a starting point for the training of women health workers.

Training opportunities for boys and men are also important, for example vocational training where former livelihoods have been destroyed.

4 Evaluation

4.1 Purpose of evaluation

Refugee programmes are expensive and so donors and aid agencies often require an evaluation. However, evaluation is an integral part of refugee health care in its own right, and should be built into the programme from the outset.

The main aim of a refugee health programme is to reduce excess mortality and morbidity and maintain both at 'acceptable' levels. Therefore the main reason for evaluating is to consider and describe the extent to which that objective has been achieved. The value and effectiveness of what has been done must be assessed in order to modify the programme if necessary, to learn from mistakes and build on strengths in ongoing programme planning.

It is important to develop specific, quantifiable objectives which relate to the main aim; for example, to reduce the under-five mortality rate by 25 per cent in six months.

4.2 Timing and scope of evaluation

Evaluation may take place at a specific point i.e. mid-way through a planned programme, or at a specific phase of the programme (formative evaluation); or at the end of the programme (summative). It may have a narrow sectoral focus (immunisation, sanitation) or include management, financial and technical aspects.

4.3 Information required for evaluation

In order to carry out a successful evaluation, which will enable lessons to be learnt, two types of information are necessary:

1 A comprehensive preliminary assessment, which has provided baseline data on a number of indicators, from which change can be measured, and identified

objectives and indicators for monitoring and evaluation.

2   Routine monitoring systems which provide reliable and relevant data.

4.4 Types of indicator

Indicators are significant variables which help to measure changes. They are evaluation tools which can measure change directly or indirectly. They can be quantitative, concerned with things that can be counted or measured, or qualitative, concerned with the quality of what is being evaluated, such as attitude and behaviour. They can be classified for purposes of health evaluation as follows:

1 Inputs

budget (capital and recurrent costs)

personnel

supplies

equipment

donations and voluntary work contributions

2 Processes

level of participation

capacity building for refugees, especially women refugees

acceptability of services, particularly to women

quality of services

attitudes of health workers

supervision and management methods and style

3 Outputs

availability (number and type of health facilities)

accessibility

uptake

coverage of services

number of trained health workers

frequency of training sessions

number and pattern of usage of water and sanitation facilities

4 Impacts

incidence and prevalence of main communicable diseases

maternal mortality rates

child mortality rates

crude mortality rates

nutritional status

prevalence of micronutrient deficiencies.

The type of evaluation will influence the choice of indicators. If it is an economic evaluation, such as a financial audit, then financial indicators will be used. If it is a cost-effectiveness evaluation, then financial indicators together with output indicators will be used. If the emphasis of the evaluation is on process, then more qualitative indicators will be used, such as refugee level of involvement, acceptability of services and activities of women.

4.5 Data collection for evaluation

Quantitative data can be in the form of written records from clinics, or specific population-based surveys of health and nutrition status or vaccination coverage. Other numerical records for use in evaluation might be the census (total count) of water distribution points, number of latrines constructed. Personnel records are also useful, such as inventory (listing) of numbers of trained health workers, number and type of training sessions held.

Qualitative data can be obtained from systematic observation of refugee meetings, noting, for example, the level of participation of women and men; systematic observation of hygiene practices at household level; or case studies of individuals or groups. Interviews can be a good source of qualitative data. These can be with key informants, or with groups. They can be based on questionnaires or use more informal techniques, such as semi-structured interviews, focus groups, and various rapid appraisal techniques, such as ranking exercises.

4.6 Participatory evaluation

Participatory evaluation methodologies, whereby the people concerned in a programme as staff or beneficiaries take a significant part in planning and carrying out the evaluation, may be appropriate for evaluating refugee health programmes. The usefulness of these will depend on the level of participation that has already been established in the programme by the health workers and community in general.

4.7 Reporting and using the evaluation findings

The evaluation report should include a statement of the objectives of the evaluation and details of what methodology was used. Written reports should be clear, and quantitative information should be presented in the form of tables with explanatory notes.

It is important that the report is produced promptly, that there is feedback, preferably on site in person, to those involved in the programme, including the refugees, and that it is distributed to all appropriate people and agencies. The report may be used in full or in an edited version to lobby for more resources or action on other issues.

The report should state recommendations for future action clearly and identify action points and areas of responsibility. Evaluation is a tool for learning to work more effectively in future.

Appendix 1: Mortality rates

Mortality rates are expressed as a number of deaths per 1,000 (or 10,000) population within a given time frame (crude mortality rate or CMR). This means that in order to calculate rates, all deaths have to be recorded and the total population of the camp has to be known, or it must be possible to estimate the total population with confidence.

During the emergency phase, when death rates are likely to be high, the CMR is usually expressed as 'number of deaths per 10,000 per day'. The following benchmarks for evaluating the seriousness of the situation are now widely accepted:

Crude Mortality Rate:

0.5 per 10,000 per day 'normal' in developing countries

<1.0 per 10,000 per day under control

>1.0 per 10,000 per day very serious situation

>2.0 per 10,000 per day out of control

>5.0 per 10,000 per day catastrophic

Young children are often severely affected by camp conditions, and death rates among under-fives are likely to show the greatest increase. If possible, under-five mortality figures should therefore be disaggregated. The benchmarks for the under-five mortality rate (< 5MR) are approximately double those of the CMR.

Under-five Mortality Rate:

<1.0 per 10,000 per day 'normal'

<2.0 per 10,000 per day under control

>2.0 per 10,000 per day very serious situation

>4.0 per 10,000 per day out of control

>10.0 per 10,000 per day catastrophic

Calculating crude mortality rates over short periods of time (less than one month)

1 Total the deaths for a given number of days.
2 Divide the total by the number of days over which data were gathered — this gives the average number of deaths per day.
3 Divide this number by the size of the displaced population.
4 Multiply by 10,000 for a **daily crude mortality rate.**
(CDC, 1992)

If the camp has been established for some time and there has been no mortality surveillance, there may be a need to conduct a retrospective mortality survey, asking a random sample of the population about deaths in the family over a given recall period. The length of recall period should not exceed six months, even if the camp has existed for longer than that, because reliability of recall will be a problem. Sample size will depend on the estimated mortality rate, recall period, and size of population. (Consult a statistician!)

Mortality is commonly under-reported, for a number of reasons; not least because a death reduces the family entitlement to food and other relief goods. It is important to make every effort to encourage reporting, for example, by providing burial cloth to relatives of the bereaved. It is also important to cross-check mortality registration reports and to complement with other systems, such as paid 24-hour grave-watchers

Appendix 2: Nutrition surveys

Planning and carrying out a formal survey requires knowledge and experience of survey design, sampling and statistics. Measuring children requires literacy, numeracy and accuracy. Experience of rural field conditions is also important, otherwise your proposed sampling methods may be impossible to apply in practice. *If you do not have these skills, think seriously before you start a survey because wrong information is even worse than no information!*

A nutrition survey estimates the rate or prevalence of malnutrition in the population. Anthropometric (body) measurements of children are used to estimate the rate of malnutrition. The prevalence of malnutrition among children in a whole population is estimated from the results of measuring a sample of children. The accuracy of these statistical estimates depends on i) correct sampling methods and ii) careful measurements.

Correct sampling methods

Having decided what to measure, you now have to decide who to measure. It is rarely possible to include everybody in the population in a survey, so to save time and money a limited number of people are chosen. The choice of people is known as sampling and the people chosen are the sample.

The characteristics of the sample should be similar to the characteristics of the total population. This is what is meant by 'a representative sample'. A sample that does not represent the population is said to be biased. For example, if mothers volunteer to have their children measured, rather than being randomly selected, this would result in a biased sample.

The different ways to obtain a sample are as follows:-

- **simple random sampling**, by e.g.picking names out of a hat or at random from a list
- **interval sampling**, by e.g. selecting every fiftieth person on a list
- **cluster sampling**, where groups of people rather than individuals are selected to comprise the sample. The sample size is equal to the number of clusters multiplied by the number of children in each cluster. Statisticians recommend **at least 24 clusters, and preferably 30 clusters** for estimating the rate of malnutrition in a population.

When the total population is included in the survey, for example, when all the children in a community are measured, it is known as a census, and is no longer a sample survey. The results of a census only apply to the population measured.

NB: — *Findings from a sample survey*

The prevalence of malnutrition in the sample is expressed as a single figure, known as the point prevalence; for example, 14.3 per cent of the children in the sample are malnourished. The results from the sample can then be used to estimate the prevalence of malnutrition in the whole population. This estimate is expressed as a range of values known as confidence limits (rather than a single figure like the point prevalence). For example, the rate of malnutrition in the population might be estimated to be between 12.3 and 21.0 per cent. The confidence limits are 12.3 and 21.0. and the confidence interval is 8.7. The confidence interval represents the probability (usually 95%) that the *true* prevalence of malnutrition in the population (as opposed to the sample) lies within the range of the confidence limits. This calculation enables comparisons to be made between the results of different surveys.

Measurements

Nutrition indices are bodily measurements related to age or height, and are used to estimate malnutrition by comparing the survey population with the norm for the healthy reference population.

An inadequate diet and/or infection may lead to weight loss. In the short term, a child suffering weight loss becomes thin or wasted. This is known as acute malnutrition, and is reflected by the nutrition indices weight for height or length (WFH/L) and mid-upper arm circumference (MUAC).

Thinness can develop very rapidly and may occur seasonally, during the 'hungry season' which is often just before the harvest. The prevalence of thinness is greatest between 12 and 24 months of age, which is when infants are often weaned. During this time dietary deficiencies are common and diarrhoeal diseases frequent. Under favourable conditions weight can be restored rapidly.

A poor diet over a longer period may cause growth failure so the child may be short for their age or stunted. This is reflected by the height for age (HFA) index. Unlike weight loss, growth failure is not necessarily reversible.

The criteria for inclusion of children in the sample are usually as follows:-

- from age 6 months or 1 year to 5 years of age (110 or 115cm in height) for WFH surveys
- from 1 year to 5 years of age (110 or 115cm in height) for MUAC surveys

Weight for height or length (WFH/L)

Weight for height is the most common anthropometric index used in nutrition surveys. An individual's height and weight are compared with those of the reference population by calculating percentage weight for height or length (% WFH/L). This is the child's weight expressed as a percentage of the average weight of children of the same height.

An individual child's weight and height measurements may also be expressed as 'Z scores'. Z scores express a child's weight as a multiple of the standard deviation (a measure of the spread of values around the mean) of the reference population, and are also known as 'standard deviation scores'. They are statistically more correct than percentages of the reference average WFH, but are a little more complicated to calculate and less easy to understand.

Mid upper arm circumference (MUAC)

Measuring MUAC is quicker than measuring both weight and height and then calculating the percentage WFH/L or Z score. Consequently, MUAC is frequently used to screen large numbers of children in search of those who may be malnourished. It may also be used for a "one-off" survey to establish nutritional statusbut is not suitable for repeated surveys over time.

MUAC may seem easier to measure than WFH, but experienced field workers have expressed concern that it is easy to make mistakes when measuring arm circumference, either by pulling the tape too tight or by leaving it loose, especially if the child is anxious and their arm is not relaxed. Despite these problems, MUAC is as good or even better than WFH/L for the identification of malnourished children. If you decide to use it, make every effort to ensure measurements are made correctly (see *How to measure children*, below).

The same terms are used to classify malnutrition however it is measured. Children are described as adequately nourished, moderately malnourished or severely malnourished. The table below gives the cut-off points for defining levels of malnutrition for the three different indices we have described. Children with kwashiorkor must be classified and counted as severely malnourished, but it is assessed by clinical signs, not by measurement. The main sign is pitting oedema of the lower limbs. The child may or may not appear thin and wasted, but will be miserable, apathetic and have no appetite.

The results of MUAC and WFH/L surveys are not comparable. When they are both measured on the same children, MUAC tends to give larger estimates of the percentage of children who are malnourished especially in the group of children less than 2 years of age.

This means that you should *always use the nutritional index that has been used for previous surveys* in the area where you are working. If in doubt consult the local Ministry of Health and previous survey reports.

	Weight for height/length		MUAC
	%WFH/L	Z score	cm
Adequately nourished	>79.9	>-1.9	>13.4
Moderately malnourished	<80 and >69.9	< -2 and > -2.9	<13.5 and >12.4
Severely malnourished	<70	< -3.0	<12.5

Classification of nutritional status

How to measure children

Three people are needed to measure the weights and heights of children. The most experienced field worker (the measuring team leader) should position the child correctly and take the readings. The second most experienced person should record the measurements on the recording form. This person should repeat the measurement out loud to check he or she heard it correctly. A third person assists the team leader to lift or position the child.

Be relaxed and friendly and reassure the children and their mothers. If one child begins to cry or becomes anxious, others will follow suit, and accurate measurements will be even more difficult to make.

Weighing and measuring is tiring. As people become tired, accuracy suffers. Ensure adequate rests and periodically double-check measurements. Weighing and measuring is disruptive. If children are to be measured it is very difficult to ask mothers any more than the most simple questions. It is preferable to separate any weighing and measuring from interviews.

Measuring weight
- Use 25kg hanging Salter or CMS scales. They are strong, reliable and provide the necessary degree of precision.
- Use a piece of rope to secure the scales to a tree, or ceiling or from a strong pole supported on the shoulders of two people. The dial should be at eye level.
- Before each weighing session check scales with a standard weight (use a stone or jerrycan of sand that you have accurately measured beforehand). In case of inaccuracies, have a spare set of scales available.

- Adjust the needle to zero. If a heavy basket is used to suspend children, hang it on the scales when you adjust them to zero.
- Place small babies and infants in either hanging pants, a sling, or local basket, and attach to the scales. Older children are able to hold on to the bar attached to the scales and lift themselves off the ground.
- Ensure that nothing is touching the child. Stand directly in front of the dial and read the measurement to the nearest 0.1kg.
- Record the weight and any noticeable signs of malnutrition.

Measuring height and length

Height and length may be measured using the same board. Measure the height of children of 85cm and above, who are able to stand. Measure the length of children less than 85cm and those who are unable to stand. When the length of a child above 85cm is measured, 1cm should be subtracted from their length to give the equivalent height measurement.

Height

- Stand the child up straight on the base of the height board. The head, back and heels should be flat against the back of the board, with heels together and eyes looking straight ahead.
- Position the head block flat against the board and slide down on to the child's head. Ensure it is level (both tape measures should show the same readings).
- Read the height measurement to the nearest 0.5cm and call it out to the person recording the data.

Length

- Position the height/length board horizontally.
- Two people should lay the child on the board, with the child's head towards the base board. The assistant measurer holds the child's head against the base of the board, with the eyes looking straight up.
- The measuring team leader adjusts the measuring block and brings it to rest flat against the soles of the child's feet (one hand holds the block and the other holds the child's ankles).
- The team leader checks the block is level and reads the measurement to the nearest 0.5cm and calls it out to the person recording the data.

The construction of a height and length board

Use wood that is smooth and has no splinters or rough edges. The three blocks of wood on the base give it greater stability when used as a length board.

It is easier to read measurements from above the measuring block than beneath it. For this reason, position the ends of the tape measures 10cm from the base board (10cm being the height of the measuring block). This means that measurements may be read from above the block rather than beneath it.

Each board should always be used with the original blockused to position the tapes. Label the board and block so they can be easily identified and always used together.

Measuring mid-upper arm circumference (MUAC)

• Only measure MUAC on children between one and five years old. A one-year-old is normally above 75cm tall, can stand or walk, and has six teeth or more.

• Use a MUAC insertion tape to measure arm circumference. The thin end slips through the opening at the wider end and the measurement is read at the point indicated by the arrows.

• Measure MUAC on the left arm.

• To find the mid-point, stand the child facing you and ask the child to bend the left arm at the elbow at a right angle and place the left hand flat on the stomach. Use the MUAC tape to measure from the tip of the shoulder to the tip of the elbow.

• Take hold of the point of the tape at the elbow and fold back on to the point on the shoulder tip. Mark with a pen the position of the fold, which is the middle point of the upper arm.

• At the mid-point, wrap the tape closely round the arm. Do not pull tightly or leave loose. Read the measurement to the nearest 0.1cm.

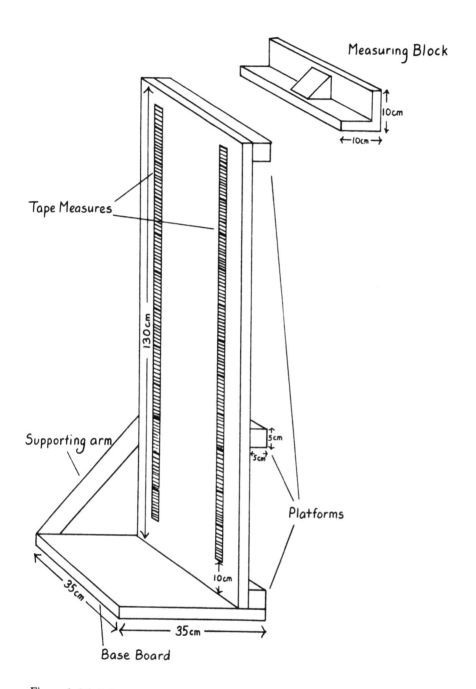

Figure 1 A height and length board

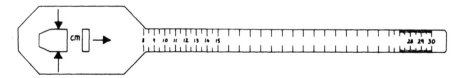

Figure2 An insertion tape

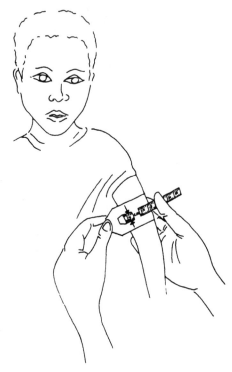

Figure3 Using an insertion tape

NB If an insertion tape is unavailable, it is perfectly possible to use an ordinary tape measure; but in this case, it is best to start the measurement at the 10cm point, which will give you the first 10cm of the tape to hold.

Table 8: Weight for length for boys and girls between 49 and 84.5cm

BOYS

LENGTH CM	-3S.D.	-2S.D.	-1S.D.	MEDIAN
49.0	2.1	2.5	2.8	3.1
49.5	2.1	2.5	2.9	3.2
50.0	2.2	2.5	2.9	3.3
50.5	2.2	2.6	3.0	3.4
51.0	2.2	2.6	3.1	3.5
51.5	2.3	2.7	3.1	3.6
52.0	2.3	2.8	3.2	3.7
52.5	2.4	2.8	3.3	3.8
53.0	2.4	2.9	3.4	3.9
53.5	2.5	3.0	3.5	4.0
54.0	2.6	3.1	3.6	4.1
54.5	2.6	3.2	3.7	4.2
55.0	2.7	3.3	3.8	4.3
55.5	2.8	3.3	3.9	4.5
56.0	2.9	3.5	4.0	4.6
56.5	3.0	3.6	4.1	4.7
57.0	3.1	3.7	4.3	4.8
57.5	3.2	3.8	4.4	5.0
58.0	3.3	3.9	4.5	5.1
58.5	3.4	4.0	4.6	5.2
59.0	3.5	4.1	4.8	5.4
59.5	3.6	4.2	4.9	5.5
60.0	3.7	4.4	5.0	5.7
60.5	3.8	4.5	5.1	5.8
61.0	4.0	4.6	5.3	5.9
61.5	4.1	4.8	5.4	6.1
62.0	4.2	4.9	5.6	6.2
62.5	4.3	5.0	5.7	6.4
63.0	4.5	5.2	5.8	6.5
63.5	4.6	5.3	6.0	6.7
64.0	4.7	5.4	6.1	6.8
64.5	4.9	5.6	6.3	7.0
65.0	5.0	5.7	6.4	7.1
65.5	5.1	5.8	6.5	7.3
66.0	5.3	6.0	6.7	7.4
66.5	5.4	6.1	6.8	7.6
67.0	5.5	6.2	7.0	7.7
67.5	5.7	6.4	7.1	7.8
68.0	5.8	6.5	7.3	8.0
68.5	5.9	6.6	7.4	8.1
69.0	6.0	6.8	7.5	8.3
69.5	6.2	6.9	7.7	8.4

GIRLS

LENGTH CM	-3S.D.	-2S.D.	-1S.D.	MEDIAN
49.0	2.2	2.6	2.9	3.3
49.5	2.2	2.6	3.0	3.4
50.0	2.3	2.6	3.0	3.4
50.5	2.3	2.7	3.1	3.5
51.0	2.3	2.7	3.1	3.5
51.5	2.4	2.8	3.2	3.6
52.0	2.4	2.8	3.3	3.7
52.5	2.5	2.9	3.4	3.8
53.0	2.5	3.0	3.4	3.9
53.5	2.6	3.1	3.5	4.0
54.0	2.7	3.1	3.6	4.1
54.5	2.7	3.2	3.7	4.2
55.0	2.8	3.3	3.8	4.3
55.5	2.9	3.4	3.9	4.4
56.0	3.0	3.5	4.0	4.5
56.5	3.0	3.6	4.1	4.6
57.0	3.1	3.7	4.2	4.8
57.5	3.2	3.8	4.3	4.9
58.0	3.3	3.9	4.4	5.0
58.5	3.4	4.0	4.6	5.1
59.0	3.5	4.1	4.7	5.3
59.5	3.6	4.2	4.8	5.4
60.0	3.7	4.3	4.9	5.5
60.5	3.8	4.4	5.1	5.7
61.0	3.9	4.6	5.2	5.8
61.5	4.0	4.7	5.3	6.0
62.0	4.1	4.8	5.4	6.1
62.5	4.2	4.9	5.6	6.2
63.0	4.4	5.0	5.7	6.4
63.5	4.5	5.2	5.8	6.5
64.0	4.6	5.3	6.0	6.7
64.5	4.7	5.4	6.1	6.8
65.0	4.8	5.5	6.3	7.0
65.5	4.9	5.7	6.4	7.1
66.0	5.1	5.8	6.5	7.3
66.5	5.2	5.9	6.7	7.4
67.0	5.3	6.0	6.8	7.5
67.5	5.4	6.2	6.9	7.7
68.0	5.5	6.3	7.1	7.8
68.5	5.6	6.4	7.2	8.0
69.0	5.8	6.5	7.3	8.1
69.5	5.9	6.7	7.5	8.2

| | **BOYS** | | | | | | **GIRLS** | | | |
LENGTH CM	-3S.D.	-2S C	-1S.D.	MEDIAN		LENGTH CM	-3S.D.	-2S.D.	-1S.D.	MEDIAN
70.0	6.3	7.0	7.8	8.5		70.0	6.0	6.8	7.6	8.4
70.5	6.4	7.2	7.9	8.7		70.5	6.1	6.9	7.7	8.5
71.0	6.5	7.3	8.1	8.8		71.0	6.2	7.0	7.8	8.6
71.5	6.7	7.4	8.2	8.9		71.5	6.3	7.1	8.0	8.8
72.0	6.8	7.5	8.3	9.1		72.0	6.4	7.2	8.1	8.9
72.5	6.9	7.7	8.4	9.2		72.5	6.5	7.4	8.2	9.0
73.0	7.0	7.8	8.6	9.3		73.0	6.6	7.5	8.3	9.1
73.5	7.1	7.9	8.7	9.5		73.5	6.7	7.6	8.4	9.3
74.0	7.2	8.0	8.8	9.6		74.0	6.8	7.7	8.5	9.4
74.5	7.3	8.1	8.9	9.7		74.5	6.9	7.8	8.6	9.5
75.0	7.4	8.2	9.0	9.8		75.0	7.0	7.9	8.7	9.6
75.5	7.5	8.3	9.1	9.9		75.5	7.1	8.0	8.8	9.7
76.0	7.6	8.4	9.2	10.0		76.0	7.2	8.1	8.9	9.8
76.5	7.7	8.5	9.3	10.2		76.5	7.3	8.2	9.0	9.9
77.0	7.8	8.6	9.4	10.3		77.0	7.4	8.3	9.1	10.0
77.5	7.9	8.7	9.5	10.4		77.5	7.5	8.4	9.2	10.1
78.0	8.0	8.8	9.7	10.5		78.0	7.6	8.5	9.3	10.2
78.5	8.1	8.9	9.8	10.6		78.5	7.7	8.6	9.4	10.3
79.0	8.2	9.0	9.9	10.7		79.0	7.8	8.7	9.5	10.4
79.5	8.2	9.1	10.0	10.8		79.5	7.9	8.7	9.6	10.5
80.0	8.3	9.2	10.1	10.9		80.0	8.0	8.8	9.7	10.6
80.5	8.4	9.3	10.1	11.0		80.5	8.0	8.9	9.8	10.7
81.0	8.5	9.4	10.2	11.1		81.0	8.1	9.0	9.9	10.8
81.5	8.6	9.5	10.3	11.2		81.5	8.2	9.1	10.0	10.9
82.0	8.7	9.6	10.4	11.3		82.0	8.3	9.2	10.1	11.0
82.5	8.8	9.6	10.5	11.4		82.5	8.4	9.3	10.2	11.1
83.0	8.8	9.7	10.6	11.5		83.0	8.5	9.4	10.3	11.2
83.5	8.9	9.8	10.7	11.6		83.5	8.6	9.5	10.4	11.3
84.0	9.0	9.9	10.8	11.7		84.0	8.7	9.6	10.5	11.4
84.5	9.1	10.0	10.9	11.8		84.5	8.7	9.6	10.6	11.5

(Source: NCHS/CDC/WHO Reference Population, from *Measuring Change in Nutritional Status*, 1983. WHO, Geneva)

Table 2 Weight for height for boys and girls between 85 and 130cm

BOYS

STATURE CM	-3S.D.	-2S.D.	-1S.D.	MEDIAN
85.0	8.9	9.9	11.0	12.1
85.5	8.9	10.0	11.1	12.2
86.0	9.0	10.1	11.2	12.3
86.5	9.1	10.2	11.3	12.5
87.0	9.2	10.3	11.5	12.6
87.5	9.3	10.4	11.6	12.7
88.0	9.4	10.5	11.7	12.8
88.5	9.5	10.6	11.8	12.9
89.0	9.6	10.7	11.9	13.0
89.5	9.7	10.8	12.0	13.1
90.0	9.8	10.9	12.1	13.3
90.5	9.9	11.0	12.2	13.4
91.0	9.9	11.1	12.3	13.5
91.5	10.0	11.2	12.4	13.6
92.0	10.1	11.3	12.5	13.7
92.5	10.2	11.4	12.6	13.9
93.0	10.3	11.5	12.8	14.0
93.5	10.4	11.6	12.9	14.1
94.0	10.5	11.7	13.0	14.2
94.5	10.6	11.8	13.1	14.3
95.0	10.7	11.9	13.2	14.5
95.5	10.8	12.0	13.3	14.6
96.0	10.9	12.1	13.4	14.7
96.5	11.0	12.2	13.5	14.8
97.0	11.0	12.4	13.7	15.0
97.5	11.1	12.5	13.8	15.1
98.0	11.2	12.6	13.9	15.2
98.5	11.3	12.7	14.0	15.4
99.0	11.4	12.8	14.1	15.5
99.5	11.5	12.9	14.3	15.6
100.0	11.6	13.0	14.4	15.7
100.5	11.7	13.1	14.5	15.9
101.0	11.8	13.2	14.6	16.0
101.5	11.9	13.3	14.7	16.2
102.0	12.0	13.4	14.9	16.3
102.5	12.1	13.6	15.0	16.4
103.0	12.2	13.7	15.1	16.6
103.5	12.3	13.8	15.3	16.7
104.0	12.4	13.9	15.4	16.9
104.5	12.6	14.0	15.5	17.0
105.0	12.7	14.2	15.6	17.1
105.5	12.8	14.3	15.8	17.3

GIRLS

STATURE CM	-3S.D.	-2S.D.	-1S.D.	MEDIAN
85.0	8.6	9.7	10.8	11.8
85.5	8.7	9.8	10.9	11.9
86.0	8.8	9.9	11.0	12.0
86.5	8.9	10.0	11.1	12.2
87.0	9.0	10.1	11.2	12.3
87.5	9.1	10.2	11.3	12.4
88.0	9.2	10.3	11.4	12.5
88.5	9.3	10.4	11.5	12.6
89.0	9.3	10.5	11.6	12.7
89.5	9.4	10.6	11.7	12.8
90.0	9.5	10.7	11.8	12.9
90.5	9.6	10.7	11.9	13.0
91.0	9.7	10.8	12.0	13.2
91.5	9.8	10.9	12.1	13.3
92.0	9.9	11.0	12.2	13.4
92.5	9.9	11.1	12.3	13.5
93.0	10.0	11.2	12.4	13.6
93.5	10.1	11.3	12.5	13.7
94.0	10.2	11.4	12.6	13.9
94.5	10.3	11.5	12.8	14.0
95.0	10.4	11.6	12.9	14.1
95.5	10.5	11.7	13.0	14.2
96.0	10.6	11.8	13.1	14.3
96.5	10.7	11.9	13.2	14.5
97.0	10.7	12.0	13.3	14.6
97.5	10.8	12.1	13.4	14.7
98.0	10.9	12.2	13.5	14.9
98.5	11.0	12.3	13.7	15.0
99.0	11.1	12.4	13.8	15.1
99.5	11.2	12.5	13.9	15.2
100.0	11.3	12.7	14.0	15.4
100.5	11.4	12.8	14.1	15.5
101.0	11.5	12.9	14.3	15.6
101.5	11.6	13.0	14.4	15.8
102.0	11.7	13.1	14.5	15.9
102.5	11.8	13.2	14.6	16.0
103.0	11.9	13.3	14.7	16.2
103.5	12.0	13.4	14.9	16.3
104.0	12.1	13.5	15.0	16.5
104.5	12.2	13.7	15.1	16.6
105.0	12.3	13.8	15.3	16.7
105.5	12.4	13.9	15.4	16.9

	BOYS						GIRLS			
STATURE CM	-3S.D.	-2S.D.	-1S.D.	MEDIAN		STATURE CM	-3S.D.	-2S.D.	-1S.D.	MEDIAN
106.0	12.9	14.4	15.9	17.4		106.0	12.5	14.0	15.5	17.0
106.5	13.0	14.5	16.1	17.6		106.5	12.6	14.1	15.7	17.2
107.0	13.1	14.7	16.2	17.7		107.0	12.7	14.3	15.8	17.3
107.5	13.2	14.8	16.3	17.9		107.5	12.8	14.4	15.9	17.5
108.0	13.4	14.9	16.5	18.0		108.0	13.0	14.5	16.1	17.6
108.5	13.5	15.0	16.6	18.2		108.5	13.1	14.6	16.2	17.8
109.0	13.6	15.2	16.8	18.3		109.0	13.2	14.8	16.4	17.9
109.5	13.7	15.3	16.9	18.5		109.5	13.3	14.9	16.5	18.1
110.0	13.8	15.4	17.1	18.7		110.0	13.4	15.0	16.6	18.2
110.5	14.0	15.6	17.2	18.8		110.5	13.6	15.2	16.8	18.4
111.0	14.1	15.7	17.4	19.0		111.0	13.7	15.3	16.9	18.6
111.5	14.2	15.9	17.5	19.1		111.5	13.8	15.5	17.1	18.7
112.0	14.4	16.0	17.7	19.3		112.0	14.0	15.6	17.2	18.9
112.5	14.5	16.1	17.8	19.5		112.5	14.1	15.7	17.4	19.0
113.0	14.6	16.3	18.0	19.6		113.0	14.2	15.9	17.5	19.2
113.5	14.8	16.4	18.1	19.8		113.5	14.4	16.0	17.7	19.4
114.0	14.9	16.6	18.3	20.0		114.0	14.5	16.2	17.9	19.5
114.5	15.0	16.7	18.5	20.2		114.5	14.6	16.3	18.0	19.7
115.0	15.2	16.9	18.6	20.3		115.0	14.8	16.5	18.2	19.9
115.5	15.3	17.1	18.8	20.5		115.5	14.9	16.6	18.4	20.1
116.0	15.5	17.2	18.9	20.7		116.0	15.0	16.8	18.5	20.3
116.5	15.6	17.4	19.1	20.9		116.5	15.2	16.9	18.7	20.4
117.0	15.8	17.5	19.3	21.1		117.0	15.3	17.1	18.9	20.6
117.5	15.9	17.7	19.5	21.2		117.5	15.5	17.3	19.0	20.8
118.0	16.1	17.9	19.6	21.4		118.0	15.6	17.4	19.2	21.0
118.5	16.2	18.0	19.8	21.6		118.5	15.8	17.6	19.4	21.2
119.0	16.4	18.2	20.0	21.8		119.0	15.9	17.7	19.6	21.4
119.5	16.6	18.4	20.2	22.0		119.5	16.1	17.9	19.8	21.6
120.0	16.7	18.5	20.4	22.2		120.0	16.2	18.1	20.0	21.8
120.5	16.9	18.7	20.6	22.4		120.5	16.4	18.3	20.1	22.0
121.0	17.0	18.9	20.7	22.6		121.0	16.5	18.4	20.3	22.2
121.5	17.2	19.1	20.9	22.8		121.5	16.7	18.6	20.5	22.5
122.0	17.4	19.2	21.1	23.0		122.0	16.8	18.8	20.7	22.7
122.5	17.5	19.4	21.3	23.2		122.5	17.0	19.0	20.9	22.9
123.0	17.7	19.6	21.5	23.4		123.0	17.1	19.1	21.1	23.1
123.5	17.9	19.8	21.7	23.6		123.5	17.3	19.3	21.3	23.4
124.0	18.0	20.0	21.9	23.9		124.0	17.4	19.5	21.6	23.6
124.5	18.2	20.2	22.1	24.1		124.5	17.6	19.7	21.8	23.9
125.0	18.4	20.4	22.3	24.3		125.0	17.8	19.9	22.0	24.1
125.5	18.6	20.5	22.5	24.5		125.5	17.9	20.1	22.2	24.3
126.0	18.7	20.7	22.8	24.8		126.0	18.1	20.2	22.4	24.6
126.5	18.9	20.9	23.0	25.0		126.5	18.2	20.4	22.7	24.9

BOYS

STATURE CM	-3S.D.	-2S.D.	-1S.D.	MEDIAN
127.0	19.1	21.1	23.2	25.2
127.5	19.2	21.3	23.4	25.5
128.0	19.4	21.5	23.6	25.7
128.5	19.6	21.7	23.8	26.0
129.0	19.8	21.9	24.1	26.2
129.5	19.9	22.1	24.3	26.5
130.0	20.1	22.3	24.5	26.8

GIRLS

STATURE CM	-3S.D.	-2S.D.	-1S.D.	MEDIAN
127.0	18.4	20.6	22.9	25.1
127.5	18.6	20.8	23.1	25.4
128.0	18.7	21.0	23.3	25.7
128.5	18.9	21.2	23.6	25.9
129.0	19.0	21.4	23.8	26.2
129.5	19.2	21.6	24.1	26.5
130.0	19.4	21.8	24.3	26.8

(Source: NCHS/CDC/WHO Reference Population, from *Measuring Change in Nutritional Status*, 1983, WHO, Geneva)

(The information in this appendix is taken from Young, H, *Food Scarcity and Famine: Assessment and Response*, Oxfam Practical Health Guide No. 7.)

Appendix 3: Nutritional values of food aid commodities

Food	Energy Kcal	Protein g	Fat g
Cereals			
Maize, white, meal	360	9.0	3.8
Millet, whole grain	315	7.4	1.3
Millet, flour	320	5.6	1.4
Rice, polished	360	7.0	0.5
Sorghum, whole grain	335	11.0	3.0
Sorghum, flour	335	9.5	2.8
Teff, whole grain	341	9.8	2.5
Wheat, whole grain	330	12.3	1.5
Wheat, flour	350	11.5	2.0
Beans, peas and lentils			
Beans, dried	335	22.0	1.5
Horse bean	342	25.0	1.5
Lentils, dried	325	25.0	1.2
Peas, dried	300	22.0	1.1
Soya beans	405	34.0	1.8
Nuts			
Groundnuts, fresh	345	19.0	6.2
Groundnuts, dried	570	23.0	45.0
Sugar	400		
Vegetable oil	900		100.0
Dried skimmed milk (DSM)	360	36.0	
Dried whole milk	490	23.5	24.0
Corn soy milk	380	18.0	6.0
Instant corn soy milk	365	12.2	4.0
Wheat soy blend	370	20.0	6.0
Oxfam food aid biscuits	465	8.6	18.0
Dried salted fish	270	47.0	7.5
Canned fish in oil	305	22.0	24.0
Dried fruit	270	4.0	0.5
Dried dates	245	2.0	0.5

Food aid biscuits

Biscuits are a luxury item for most people and not a regular part of the diet. Most biscuits are expensive and are not a good source of nutrition. For these reasons the distribution of biscuits is inappropriate except in certain circumstances.

Food Aid biscuits provide instant energy and other nutrients. The Oxfam biscuit is one example, being high in energy and rich in protein. One packet of six biscuits contains 520Kcal and 9.6gm protein and at least half of the WHO/FAO recommended daily intakes of certain vitamins and minerals. Unlike other foods that might be available, biscuits need no cooking and no careful measuring or preparation before eating. In the early stages of a sudden emergency, when people are without food or the equipment and fuel for its preparation, the distribution of food aid biscuits provides immediate nourishment and can make all the difference to people's morale, and gives them confidence that help is being organised.

The biscuits' main functions are for short-term supplementary feeding, until other alternatives can be established and as part of a therapeutic feeding programme. Severely malnourished children often lose their appetite but may be coaxed to eat again by having a biscuit to suck. Biscuits are sometimes useful for the night feed, as fewer staff are available for preparation of food or supervision of feeding.

(The information in this appendix is taken from Young, H, *Food Scarcity and Famine: Assessment and Response*, Oxfam Practical Health Guide No. 7.)

Appendix 4: Vitamin and mineral deficiencies

Vitamin and mineral deficiencies are caused by a lack of essential minerals or vitamins in the diet. They may cause permanent damage to health and even death.

In times of food scarcity and famine, the most important deficiency disease is xerophthalmia — vitamin A deficiency — which can cause permanent blindness and may also contribute to increased incidence, severity and duration of infectious diseases such as measles, diarrhoea and respiratory tract infections.

Where people are totally dependent on food aid rations, other deficiency diseases may also develop, for example, scurvy (vitamin C deficiency), pellagra (niacin deficiency) or nutritional anaemias (iron or folic acid deficiency).

To assess if vitamin deficiencies might be a problem look for the danger signs listed below:

- Total dependence on food rations which are low in essential vitamins and minerals.
- A previous period of hardship: failed harvest, which means a prolonged hungry season; travelling for several weeks; destitution and limited access to food.
- A switch from lightly milled local cereals or a diet based on animal products, to highly refined cereals, such as white flour or polished rice.
- A lack of green leafy vegetables, unmilled cereals and dried peas and beans in local markets.
- A maize-based diet low in protein.
- Evidence of protein energy malnutrition.

Actions to treat and prevent vitamin deficiencies should be taken if any of these danger signs exist. Do not wait until a proper survey to estimate the prevalence of vitamin deficiencies is completed.

IF THE FIRST TWO DANGER SIGNS ARE PRESENT, DISTRIBUTE VITAMIN A TO ALL CHILDREN AGED FIVE AND BELOW. Vitamin A deficiency can be prevented by a one-off distribution of vitamin A capsules every six months. It is not possible to give similar protection against other deficiencies, because the other vitamins are not stored in the body and must be consumed on a daily basis. Distribution of vitamin pills on a regular basis to a large population is impractical; it is logistically difficult, culturally inappropriate and requires vast quantities of pills and a well established distribution network. Instead, consider the following options for prevention:

- Distribute foods containing the essential nutrients.
- Distribute a larger ration to allow trading in local markets for more nutritious foods.
- Distribute fortified foods to the most vulnerable groups, such as, fortified biscuits; fortified dried skimmed milk as part of a porridge pre-mix or prepared under supervision; or fortified cereal-legume pre-mixes (Corn Soy Milk).
- Support home and community gardens by providing tools and seeds and supporting demonstration plots.

Vitamin A deficiency — xerophthalmia

If not recognised and treated, vitamin A deficiency can lead to permanent blindness. Measles may be more severe and of longer duration among children with vitamin A deficiency and is associated with a higher risk of mortality. Measles contributes to post-illness malnutrition and will rapidly deplete stores of vitamin A. Treatment with high doses of vitamin A is therefore vital. The most important target groups are those who show signs of deficiency, those with infectious diseases, and those suffering from malnutrition.

Communities affected by food scarcity and famine are at risk of developing vitamin A deficiency. In these situations prevention of vitamin A deficiency is essential. Large doses of vitamin A should be administered to all children under six years old. Supplementation doses of vitamin A to prevent deficiency are as follows:

Children over 1 year and under 6 years	200,000 IU orally every 3 to 6 months
Infants 6 - 12 months and older children who weigh less than 8 kg.	100,000 IU orally every 3 to 6 months
Lactating mothers	200,000 IU orally once at delivery or during the next 2 months.

200,000 IU = 60,000mg retinol

There are two main forms of vitamin A: retinol (preformed vitamin A), and beta carotene (an orange or red pigment found in fruits and vegetables), which the human body converts to vitamin A. The biological activity of vitamin A is expressed as Retinol Equivalents (RE):

77

1 KE = 1 µg retinol or 6 µg beta carotene.

The biological activity of vitamin A may also be expressed as International Units (IU); 1 I.U. = 0.3 µg retinol.

Daily requirements: (FAO/WHO recommended requiremnts)

Retinol equivalents
µg/day

Infants	350
Pregnant women	600
Lactating women	850

Supplementation: Supplementation with 200,000 IU vitamin A will give protection or from 3 to 6 months.

Food sources: Green leafy vegetables, deep yellow or orange fruits and vegetables, red palm oil, fortified margarine, whole milk, liver, dairy products. Fortified dried skimmed milk (1500 µg per 100 g dry weight). Corn soy milk (500 µg per 100 g dry weight).

Lead time: Vitamin A is stored in the liver and there may be a delay of several months before signs of deficiency show.

Signs and symptoms of deficiency: Night blindness — unable to see in poor light (after sunset, inside huts), while those with normal sight are able to see well. Mothers may know that the night vision of their child is poor.
Conjunctival xerosis — Areas on the white surface of the eyeball (conjunctive) become dry and dull.
Bitots spots — Foamy patches at the sides of the eye.
Corneal xerosis and ulceration — The central transparent part of the eye (cornea) becomes cloudy, followed by ulceration.
Keratomalacia — The cornea may burst leading to loss of the eye contents and blindness.

Treatment of xerophthalmia:

Adult males, and children over 1 year: On diagnosis 200,000 IU vitamin A orally. The following day 200,000 IU vitamin A orally. Four weeks later 200,000 IU vitamin A orally.

Children under 1 year and children of any age who weigh less than 8kg: Treat with half doses shown above.

Women of reproductive age, pregnant or not: For night blindness or Bitots spots treat with a daily dose of 100,000 IU daily for 2 weeks.

For children with complicated measles: 200 000 IU vitamin A orally on day 1.
200 000 IU vitamin A orally on day 2.

Vitamin C deficiency — scurvy

Refugees in camps in Somalia and Ethiopia and displaced people in Sudan have suffered from scurvy as a result of dependency on food rations low in vitamin C.

Daily requirements: 10 - 35mg daily in diet e.g. small tomato or leafy vegetable.

Food sources: Fresh fruits and vegetables, breast milk.

Lead time: Between 2-3 months.

Signs and symptoms: Scurvy is recognised by swollen and bleeding gums leading to loss of teeth and/or swollen, painful joints (in particular the hips and knees) that reduce mobility. Internal haemorrhaging can lead to death. Risk of mortality among pregnant women giving birth is greater if they are deficient in vitamin C.

Treatment: 300mg or more daily until recovery. A diet with plentyof fresh fruit and vegetables.

Thiamine deficiency — beriberi

This occurs where people have to exist on a starchy staple food such as cassava, or highly refined cereals like white polished rice. It has been found among refugees dependent on food rations.

Daily requirements: 1mg thiamine daily in diet (0.4mg per 1000Kcal).

Food sources: Dried peas and beans, whole grain or lightly milled cereals, groundnuts, oilseeds. Destroyed by cooking.

Lead time: 12 weeks.

Signs and symptoms: Several forms exist:

Moderate deficiency — loss of appetite, malaise and weakness, especially in the legs. This may last several months.

Dry beriberi — which may lead to paralysis of the limbs.
Wet beriberi — swelling of the body (oedema) and heart failure in infants, may cause sudden death.

Treatment: 50mg thiamine followed by 10mg daily until recovery.

Niacin deficiency — pellagra

Pellagra is endemic where people eat a maize based diet with little protein rich food. It is not associated with times of food scarcity and famine, although major outbreaks have occurred recently among refugees in Zimbabwe and Malawi.

Daily intake: 15 - 20mg niacin (6.6mg per 1,000Kcal). The niacin in maize is not all biologically available.

Food sources: Whole grain cereals, groundnuts, dried peas and beans, milk. Niacin is destroyed by long cooking.

Lead time: 2 to 3 months.

Signs and symptoms: It is characterised by a skin rash on those parts of the body exposed to sunlight (dermatitis). It can cause diarrhoea and dementia.

Treatment: 50 - 100mg of niacin orally daily until skin lesions recover (usually only a few days).

Anaemia

Anaemia is a low level of haemoglobin in the blood, which affects a person's ability to make sustained physical effort. Common symptoms are general fatigue, breathlessness and giddiness. The main causes are parasitic infections (particularly hookworm); low intake or poor absorption of iron and folic acid; the need to produce new blood cells (recovery from malnutrition, or malaria).
Anaemia is common among women and children in camp situations, particularly women who are pregnant or recently delivered.

Daily intake: Iron 10 - 28mg; Folic acid 200ug. Pregnant and lactating women should be given supplements from the fourth month of pregnancy; 120mg iron, and 0.2mg folic acid per day until the birth.

Food sources: Iron: dark green leaves, meat. Diets lacking in vitamin C and/or high in fibre reduce iron absorption.
Folic acid: dark green leafy vegetables, liver and kidney. Folic acid is destroyed by

prolonged cooking.

Signs and symptoms: The tongue, finger nails or inside of the lower eyelid appear very pale. Children with severe anaemia are tired and listless and have a rapid pulse. Malnourished people are often anaemic.

Treatment: Adults: 200 - 250mg of ferrous sulphate in tablet form three times a day for at least 2 months. Children: 50mg ferrous sulphate mixture (liquid) diluted with water per day for each year of age. Treat any non-dietary causes of anaemia, such as hookworm or bleeding.

Iodine deficiency — goitre and cretinism

Iodine deficiency causes enlargement of the thyroid gland (goitre) and reproductive failure. Children born to women deficient in iodine may suffer greater or lesser degrees of mental impairment (cretinism). Goitre is rarely seen in young children.

Simple goitre, where the gland is just visible and palpable, are found in all parts of the world but do not usually affect health. Iodine deficiency is most severe in poor, isolated inland communities where the soil is deficient in iodine. Some foods, for example, cabbages (brassica) and cassava, contain goitrogenic substances which interfere with the availability of iodine to the thyroid gland.

A relief programme may provide an opportunity to raise the problem of goitre as an issue to be dealt with, even though its direct cause was not due to the immediate problem of food scarcity and famine.

Daily intake: 100–150μg daily. 2ml iodised oil (475mg/ml)given orally is sufficient for up to 2 years.

Food source: Animal products, marine fish. Where the soil lacks iodine, the food grown will be deficient in iodine.

Treatment: A simple goitre rarely requires treatment. In time, with a good diet or with a diet supplemented with iodine, it will become smaller.
(For more details, see *Controlling Iodine Deficiency Disorders in Developing Countries:* Oxfam Practical Health Guide 5.)

(The information in this appendix is taken from Young, H, *Food Scarcity and Famine: Assessment and Response*, Oxfam Practical Health Guide No. 7.)

Appendix 5: Supplementary feeding recipes

Wherever possible, base your recipes on locally available foods, such as the local cereal, peas, beans or lentils and oil. Local foods may be used to show how to prepare nutritious weaning foods that cause malnourished children to gain weight. Imported foods may encourage people to think that imported foods are 'better'.

The amount of energy, protein and fat in the following recipes was calculated using the table in Appendix 8: The nutrient content of some common foods. The recipes given below meet the recommendations in Section 4.3 about the nutritional composition of foods used as food supplements: above 20 per cent of total energy from fat and about 12 per cent of total energy from protein.

Quantities of ingredients in the recipes are given in weights, which are more accurate than using volumes. However, scales are not always available and so volume measures must be used.

Dried milk powder	650g – 750g
Dried milk powder (granules)	350g – 400g
Millet, Rice, Wheat grain, Sorghum	710g – 860g
Wheat flour	550g – 600g
Bean flour	850g
Chickpeas, split peas, kidney beans, lentils	800g – 900g
Groundnuts, soya beans, butter beans	700g – 800g
Oil	900g – 950g
Sugar	900g – 950g

The approximate weight of one litre volume of foods

Label all containers used for measuring volumes so they are used correctly. The volume of some ingredients, such as dried milk powder, varies with different brands. Always check new ingredients to see if their weight volume ratio differs.

Malted grain

Porridge made with flour from malted grain is more **energy dense** than porridge made with ordinary flour. This is because flour from malted grain does not thicken as much when cooked and so less water is needed to make a porridge of the same thickness. Malted grain has been dampened to allow it to germinate, then sun dried and milled into flour. This is a common practice in Africa.

Important rules

● Only use **safe water** – safe, piped water or water that has either been boiled and cooled or has been adequately chlorinated.

● Keep to the recipes – if you change them, make sure that fat still provides more than 20 per cent of total energy and protein about 12 per cent total energy.

● The calculation of the amount needed in the recipes is based on servings of 300mls of ready to eat food, which is all most small children are able to eat at one time.

● Keep the kitchen area clean and tidy and teach basic hygiene to the staff.

● The storage life of pre-mix is two weeks if kept in a clean, covered container. Prepared milk and porridge should never be kept longer than a few hours.

RECIPE 1: Porridge based on local ingredients

	Weight g	Energy Kcal	Protein g	Fat g
Sorghum flour	400	1340	44	12
Bean flour	200	670	44	3
Oil	100	900	-	100
Onion	50	19	-	-
Total weight	750	2929	88	115
Composition of 100g	100	390	12	15
Per cent of total energy:			12%	35%

To calculate quantities:

Quantity	6L	15L
Number of 300ml servings	20	50
Sorghum flour	860g	2.2kg
Bean flour	430g	1.1kg
Onion	60g	0.3kg
Oil	115g	0.55kg
Water	4.5L	11.2L

(one part of porridge mix to approximately 3 parts water)

Preparation: The bean flour is made from dried beans ground to a fine powder. Mix the bean flour to a smooth paste with some of the **safe** cold water. Add some more water. Bring to the boil and cook gently with the chopped onion. When nearly cooked, add the sorghum flour and stir well until cooked. Stir in the oil. The amount of water needed depends on how much the beans and flour will absorb.

(This recipe has been adapted from the recipes in: Cameron, M. and Hofvander, Y. (1983), *Manual on Feeding Infants and Young Children*, Oxford: Oxford University Press. This book contains numerous recipes based on locally available ingredients. The next three recipes are based on those found in: *Selective Feeding, Oxfam Practical Health Guide 1* and have all been successfully used in feeding programmes.)

RECIPE 2: Porridge based on a locally available flour and dried skimmed milk (DSM)

	Weight g	Energy Kcal	Protein g	Fat g
Pre-mix				
Maize flour	500	1800	45	19
Sugar	125	500	-	-
Dried skimmed milk	250	900	90	-
Oil	200	1800	-	200
Total weight	1075	5000	140	219
Composition of 100g	100	465	13	20
Percent of total energy:			11%	39%

To calculate quantities:

Amount of prepared porridge	3L	15L
Number of 300ml servings	10	50
Amount of pre-mix	750g	3.75kg
Maize flour	350g	1.75kg
Sugar	90g	0.44kg
DSM	175g	0.87kg
Oil	140g	0.70kg
Water	2.25L	11.25L

(one part pre-mix to three parts water)

To prepare pre-mix: Stir dry ingredients together until well mixed through.

To prepare porridge from pre-mix: Add enough **safe** cold water to the pre-mix to mix to a smooth paste. Gradually stir in the rest of the water. Bring to the boil and stir continuously until it is smooth and thick. Where large quantities are prepared the porridge may burn on the bottom of the pan. To prevent this bring the water to the boil before adding the water-pre-mix paste and stir until it is smooth and thick.

RECIPE 3: Porridge based on Corn Soya Milk (CSM)

	Weight g	Energy Kcal	Protein g	Fat g
Pre-mix				
Corn Soya Milk	550	2090	99	33
Sugar	100	400	-	-
Oil	100	900	-	100
Total weight	750	3390	99	133
Composition of 100g	100	452	13	18
Per cent of total energy:			12%	35%

To calculate quantities:

Quantity of prepared porridge	3L	18L
Number of 300ml servings	10	60
Amount of pre-mix	750g	4.5kg
Corn Soya Milk	550g	3.3kg
Sugar	100g	0.6kg
Oil	100g	0.6kg
Water	2.25L	13.5L

(One part pre-mix to three parts water)

Prepare as for recipe 2.

Corn Soya Milk (CSM) is a blend of cereal flour, beans and DSM and fortified with vitamins and minerals. CSM is an American food aid commodity. Other cereal legume porridge mixes may be substituted for CSM. For example *faffa* is a similar porridge mix produced in Ethiopia.

RECIPE 4: High energy milk

	Weight g	Energy Kcal	Protein g	Fat g
Pre-mix				
Sugar	250	1000	-	-
Dried skimmed milk	420	1512	151	-
Oil	320	2880	-	320
Total weight	990	5392	151	320
Composition of 100g	100	545	15	32
Per cent of total energy:			11%	53%

To calculate quantities:

Quantity of prepared milk	6L	15L
Number of 300ml servings	20	50
Amount of pre-mix	1.2kg	3kg
Dried skimmed milk	510g	1.3kg
Sugar	300g	0.8kg
Oil	390g	1.0kg
Water	4.8L	12L

(one part pre-mix plus four parts water)

Prepare as for Recipe 2.

High energy milk should only be prepared under the strictest supervision with particular attention to hygiene, as it is an ideal medium for bacteria to grow in. Discard any left over milk or porridge and **never** keep it over night. High energy milk is an excellent food for treatment of malnourished children. **Do not reduce the amount of oil.**

(The information in this appendix is taken from Young, H, *Food Scarcity and Famine: Assessment and Response*, Oxfam Practical Health Guide No. 7.)

Appendix 6: Water quality and chlorination

WHO's rural water standards are based on 'faecal indicators' (the degree of faecal contamination of water), measured by the number of coliforms per 100 ml:

0 coliforms per 100ml: ideal

0-10 coliforms per 100ml: acceptable

>10 coliforms per 100ml: not acceptable, although other factors may have to be taken into account

Whether or not chlorination is possible depends on turbidity (suspended solid matter). If turbidity is too high, it is not possible to chlorinate water effectively, because chlorine attaches itself to suspended solids and is rendered ineffective. Only water which appears fairly clear to the naked eye is suitable for treatment by chlorination. In technical terms, water should contain <5 turbidity units of suspended solids. In addition, the pH should preferably be between 7.0 and 8.0.

The amount of chlorine needed to make a given volume of water safe for consumption is the amount which gives a 'residual' of 0.2 — 0.4 mg/litre. The residual can be measured by a simple pool tester.

Water testing

In an emergency, *it is important to test water regularly*. Although in urban or industrial areas, water could be contaminated by chemicals (eg nitrates, heavy metals), this type of contamination is not usually a problem in rural areas, where refugee camps are most commonly located, and the number of substances involved make it too costly and impractical to test for chemicals routinely. In rural areas, it is sufficient to test sanitary and bacteriological parameters. In situations where no local water-testing facilities are available, the Oxfam Del Agua water-testing kit can be used. It tests for faecal contamination and a number of physical and chemical properties, including turbidity, pH, and chlorine.

Appendix 7: Drugs and equipment

This list of drugs and equipment is from *The New Emergency Health Kit*. The Basic Unit is for PHC workers'use; it contains only one antibiotic, and no injectable drugs. The Supplementary Unit is for use by doctors and medical assistants.

Basic unit (for 1000 persons for 3 months)

Drugs

Acetylsalicylic acid, tab 300 mg	3000
Aluminium hydroxide, tab 500 mg	1000
Benzyl benzoate, lotion 25%, bottle 1 litre	1
Chlorhexidine (5%), bottle 1 litre	1
Chloroquine, tab 150 mg base	2000
Ferrous sulphate + folic acid, tab 200 + 0.25 mg	2000
Gentian violet, powder, 25 g	4
Mebendazole, tab 100 mg	500
ORS (oral rehydration salts), sachet for 1 litre	200
Paracetamol, tab 100 mg	1000
Sulfamethoxazole + Trimethoprim, tab 400 + 80 mg	2000
Tetracycline eye ointment 1%, tube 5 g	50

Renewable supplies

Absorbent cotton wool, kg	1
Adhesive tape 2.5 cm × 5 m, roll	30
Bar of soap (100–200 g), bar	10
Elastic bandage (crepe) 7.5 cm × 10 m, roll	20
Gauze bandage 7.5 cm × 10 m, roll	100
Gauze compresses 10 × 10 cm, 12 ply, nonsterile	500
Ballpen, blue or black	10
Exercise book A4	4
Health care + plastic sachet	500
Small plastic bag for drugs	2000
Notepad A6	10
Thermometer (oral/rectal) Celsius/Fahrenheit	6
Protective glove, nonsterile, disposable	100
Treatment guidelines for basic list	2

Oxytoxics

Ergometrine maleate, inj. 0.2 mg/ml, 1 ml	200

Psychotherapeutic drugs

Chlorpromazine, inj. 25 mg/ml, 2 ml	20

Equipment

Nail brush, plastic, autoclavable	2
Bucket, plastic, approx. 20 litres	1
Gallipot, stainless steel, 100 ml	1
Kidney dish, stainless steel, approx. 26×14 cm	1
Dressing set (3 instruments + box)	2
Dressing tray, stainless steel, approx. $30 \times 15 \times 3$ cm	1
Drum for compresses approx. 15 cm H, Ø 14 cm	2
Foldable jerrycan, 20 litres	1
Forceps Kocher, no teeth, 12–14 cm	2
Plastic bottle, 1 litre	3
Syringe Luer, disposable, 10 ml	1
Plastic bottle, 125 ml	1
Scissors straight/blunt (12–14 cm)	2

Supplementary unit (for 10 000 persons for 3 months)

Drugs

Anaesthesics

Ketamine, inj. 50 mg/ml, 10 ml	25
Lignocaine, inj. 1%, 20 ml	50

Analgesics

Pentazocine, inj. 30 mg/ml, 1 ml	50
Probenecid, tab 500 mg	500

Anti-allergics

Dexamethasone, inj. 4 mg/ml, 1 ml	50
Prednisolone, tab 5 mg	100
Epinephrine (adrenaline), see "respiratory tract"	

Anti-epileptics

Diazepam, inj. 5 mg/ml, 2 ml	200
Phenobarbitone, tab 50 mg	1000

Anti-infective drugs

Ampicillin, tab 250 mg	2000
Ampicillin, inj. 500 mg/vial	200
Benzathine benzylpenicillin, inj. 2.4 MIU/vial	50
Chloramphenicol, caps 250 mg	2000
Chloramphenicol, inj. 1 g/vial	500
Metronidazole, tab 250 mg	2000
Nystatin, non-coated tablet, 100 000 IU	2000
Phenoxymethylpenicillin, tab 250 mg	4000
Procaine benzylpenicillin, inj. 3–4 MU/vial	1000
Quinine, inj. 300 mg/ml, 2 ml	100
Quinine sulphate, tab 300 mg	3000
Sulfadoxine + pyrimethamine, tab 500 + 25 mg	300
Tetracycline, caps or tab 250 mg	2000

Blood, drugs affecting the
  Folic acid, tab 1 mg   5000
Cardiovascular drugs
  Methyldopa, tab 250 mg   500
  Hydralazine, inj. 20 mg/ml, 1 ml   20
Dermatological drugs
  Polyvidone iodine 10%, sol., bottle 500 ml   4
  Zinc oxyde 10% ointment, kg   2
  Benzoic acid 6% + salicylic acid 3% ointment, kg   1
Diuretics
  Frusemide, inj. 10 mg/ml, 2 ml   20
  Frusemide, tab 40 mg   200
Gastrointestinal drugs
  Promethazine, tab 25 mg   500
  Promethazine, inj. 25 mg/ml, 2 ml   50
  Atropine, inj. 1 mg/ml, 1 ml   50

Respiratory tract, drugs acting on
  Aminophylline, tab 100 mg   1000
  Aminophylline, inj. 25 mg/ml, 10 ml   50
  Epinephrine (adrenaline), inj. 1 mg/ml, 1 ml   50
Solutions correcting water, electrolyte and
acid-base disturbances
  Compound solution of sodium lactate inj. sol.,   200
    with giving set and needle, 500 ml/bag
  Glucose, inj. sol. 5%, giving set and needle,   100
    500 ml/bag
  Glucose, inj. sol. 50%, 50 ml   20
  Water for injection, 10 ml/plastic vial   2000
Vitamins
  Retinol (vitamin A), caps 200 000 IU   4000
  Ascorbic acid, tab 250 mg   4000

Renewable supplies
Scalp vein infusion set, disposable, 25G (Ø 0.5 mm   300
Scalp vein infusion set, disposable, 21G (Ø 0.8 mm)   100
IV placement canula, disposable, 18G (Ø 1.7 mm)   15
IV placement canula, disposable, 22G (Ø 0.9 mm)   15
Needle Luer IV, disposable, 19G (Ø 1.1 mm × 38 mm)   1000
Needle Luer IM, disposable, 21G (Ø 0.8 mm × 40 mm)   2000
Needle Luer SC, disposable, 25G (Ø 0.5 mm × 16 mm)   100
Spinal needle, disposable, 20G (64 mm – Ø 0.9 mm)   30
Spinal needle, disposable, 23G (64 mm – Ø 0.7 mm)   30
Syringe Luer resterilizable, nylon, 2 ml   20
Syringe Luer resterilizable, nylon, 5 ml   100
Syringe Luer resterilizable, nylon, 10 ml   40
Syringe Luer, disposable, 2 ml   400
Syringe Luer, disposable, 5 ml   500
Syringe Luer, disposable, 10 ml   200
Syringe conic connector (for feeding), 60 ml   20
Feeding tube, CH5 (premature baby), disposable   20

Feeding tube, CH8, disposable	50
Feeding tube, CH16, disposable	10
Urinary catheter (Foley), no 12, disposable	10
Urinary catheter (Foley), no 14, disposable	5
Urinary catheter (Foley), no 18, disposable	5
Surgical gloves sterile and resterilizable no 6.5, pair	50
Surgical gloves sterile and resterilizable no 7.5, pair	150
Surgical gloves sterile and resterilizable no 8.5, pair	50
Sterilization test tape (for autoclave), roll	2
Chloramine, tabs or powder, kg	3
Thermometer (oral/rectal) dual Celsius/Fahrenheit	10
Spare bulb for otoscope	2
Batteries R6 alkaline AA size (for otoscope)	6
Urine collecting bag with valve, 2000 ml	10
Finger stall 2 fingers, disposable	300
Suture, synthetic absorbable, braided, size DEC.2	24
(000) with cutting needle curved 3/8, 20 mm triangular	
Suture, synthetic absorbable, braided, size DEC.3	36
(00) with cutting needle curved 3/8, 30 mm triangular	
Surgical blade (surgical knives) no 22 for handle no 4	50
Razor blade	100
Tongue depressor (wooden, disposable)	100
Gauze roll 90 m × 0.90 m	3
Gauze compresses, 10 × 10 cm, 12 ply, sterile	1000

Equipment

Clinical stethoscope, dual cup	2
Obstetrical stethoscope (metal)	1
Sphygmomanometer (adult)	1
Razor non disposable	2
Scale for adult	1
Scale hanging 25 kg × 100 g (Salter type) + 3 trousers	3
Tape measure	5
Drum for compresses, h : 15 cm, Ø 14 cm	2
Otoscope + disposable set of paediatric speculums	1
Tourniquet	2
Dressing tray, stainless steel, approx. 30 × 15 × 3 cm	1
Kidney dish, stainless steel, approx. 26 × 14 cm	1
Scissors straight/blunt, 12/14 cm	2
Forceps Kocher no teeth, 12/14 cm	2
Abscess/suture set (7 instruments + box)	2
Dressing set (3 instruments + box)	5
Pressure sterilizer, 7.5 litres (type: Prestige 7506, double rack, ref. UNIPAC 01.571.00)	1
Additional rack PHC 2 ml/5 ml, ref. Prestige 7531	2
Pressure sterilizer, 20–40 litres with basket (type UNIPAC 01.560.00)	1
Kerosene stove, single burner (type UNIPAC 01.700.00)	2
Water filter with candles, 10/20 litres (type UNIPAC 56.199.02)	3
Nail brush, plastic, autoclavable	2
Portable weight/height chart (UNIPAC 01.455.70)	1
Clinical guidelines (diagnostic and treatment manual)	2

Appendix 8: Treatment protocols for diarrhoea, fever (including malaria), and acute respiratory infections

Treatment should follow correct diagnosis. Where clinical expertise and laboratory facilities are limited, as in most refugee situations, clear case-definitions must be established and consistently followed.

For some diseases, for example, measles, the clinical picture alone allows confident diagnosis; whereas others have to be confirmed by laboratory investigation. Even then, case-definitions identifying cardinal signs and symptoms are important to allow presumptive diagnosis, especially when prompt treatment is life-saving, for example, in acute lower respiratory-tract infection in children with cough (respiratory rate faster than 50 per minute) or cholera (severe, profuse, watery diarrhoea in a person over five years of age, with or without vomiting).

Treatment protocols are essential for effective curative health care. They should constitute effective treatment, be standardised, and clearly understood by health personnel.

The sources of the treatment protocols given in this appendix are as follows:
Treatment of diarrhoea: WHO (1989) *The Treatment and Prevention of Acute Diarrhoea — Practical Guidelines* and WHO *A Manual for the Treatment of Diarrhoea*
Treatment of fever and respiratory tract infections: WHO, *The New Emergency Health Kit*

Treatment of diarrhoea

HOW TO ASSESS YOUR PATIENT

		FOR DEHYDRATION A	FOR DEHYDRATION B	FOR DEHYDRATION C	FOR OTHER PROBLEMS
1 ASK ABOUT	DIARRHOEA	Less than 4 liquid stools per day	4 to 10 liquid stools per day	More than 10 liquid stools per day	Longer than 14 days duration. Blood in the stool
	VOMITING	None or a small amount	Some	Very frequent	
	THIRST	Normal	Greater than normal	Unable to drink	
	URINE	Normal	A small amount, dark	No urine for 6 hours	
2 LOOK AT	CONDITION	Well, alert	Unwell, sleepy or irritable	Very sleepy, unconscious, floppy or having fits	Severe undernutrition
	TEARS	Present	Absent	Absent	
	EYES	Normal	Sunken	Very dry and sunken	
	MOUTH and TONGUE	Wet	Dry	Very dry	
	BREATHING	Normal	Faster than normal	Very fast and deep	
3 FEEL	SKIN	A pinch goes back quickly	A pinch goes back slowly	A pinch goes back very slowly	
	PULSE	Normal	Faster than normal	Very fast, weak or you cannot feel it	
	FONTANELLE (in infants)	Normal	Sunken	Very sunken	
4 TAKE TEMPERATURE					Fever – 38.5°C (or 101°F) or greater
5 WEIGH IF POSSIBLE		Loss of less than 25 grams for each kilogram of weight	Loss of 25-100 grams for each kilogram of weight	Loss of more than 100 grams for each kilogram of weight	
6 DECIDE		The patient has no signs of dehydration. **Use Plan A**	If the patient has 2 or more of these signs, he has **some** dehydration. **Use Plan B**	If the patient has 2 or more of these danger signs, he has **severe dehydration**. **Use Plan C**	

IF YOUR PATIENT HAS:	THEN:
Blood in the stool and diarrhoea for less than 14 days	Treat with an appropriate oral antibiotic for shigella dysentery. If this child is also – dehydrated, – severely undernourished, or – less than 1 year of age, reassess the child's progress in 24 - 48 hours. For the severely undernourished child, also refer for treatment of severe undernutrition.
Diarrhoea for longer than 14 days with or without blood	Continue feeding and refer for treatment.
Severe undernutrition	
Fever – 38.5°C (or 101°F) or greater	Show the mother how to cool the child with a wet cloth and fanning. Look for and treat other causes (for example, pneumonia, malaria).

93

TREATMENT PLAN A
TO TREAT DIARRHOEA

EXPLAIN THE THREE RULES FOR TREATING DIARRHOEA AT HOME:

1. GIVE YOUR CHILD MORE FLUIDS THAN USUAL TO PREVENT DEHYDRATION. SUITABLE FLUIDS INCLUDE:
   - The recommended home fluid or food-based fluids, such as gruel, soup, or rice water.
   - Breast milk or milk feeds prepared with twice the usual amount of water.

2. GIVE YOUR CHILD FOOD:
   - Give freshly prepared foods. Recommended foods are mixes of cereal and beans, or cereal and meat or fish. Add a few drops of oil to the food, if possible.
   - Give fresh fruit juices or bananas to provide potassium.
   - Offer food every 3 or 4 hours (6 times a day) or more often for very young children.
   - Encourage the child to eat as much as he or she wants.
   - Cook and mash or grind food well so it will be easier to digest.
   - After the diarrhoea stops, give one extra meal each day for a week, or until the child has regained normal weight.

3. TAKE YOUR CHILD TO THE HEALTH WORKER IF THE CHILD HAS ANY OF THE FOLLOWING:
   - passes many stools ⎫
   - is very thirsty ⎬ These 3 signs suggest your child is dehydrated.
   - has sunken eyes ⎭
   - has a fever
   - does not eat or drink normally
   - seems not to be getting better.

TEACH THE MOTHER HOW TO USE ORS SOLUTION AT HOME, IF:

   - The mother cannot come back if the diarrhoea gets worse.
   - It is national policy to give ORS to all children who see a health worker for diarrhoea treatment, or
   - Her child has been on Plan B, to prevent dehydration from coming back.

SHOW HER HOW TO MIX AND GIVE ORS.

SHOW HER HOW MUCH TO GIVE:
   - 50-100 ml (¼ to ½ large cup) of ORS solution after each stool for a child under 2 years old.
   - 100-200 ml (½ to 1 large cup) for older children.
   - Adults should drink as much as they want.

TELL HER IF THE CHILD VOMITS, wait 10 minutes. Then continue giving the solution but more slowly — a spoonful every 2-3 minutes.

GIVE HER ENOUGH PACKETS FOR 2 DAYS.

Note: While a child is getting ORS, he or she should be given breast milk or dilute milk feeds and should be offered food. Food-based fluids or a salt and sugar solution should *NOT* be given in addition to ORS.

EXPLAIN HOW SHE CAN PREVENT DIARRHOEA BY:

Giving only breast milk for the first 4-6 months and continuing to breast-feed for at least the first year.

Introducing clean, nutritious weaning foods at 4-6 months.

Giving her child freshly prepared and well-cooked food and clean drinking-water.

Having all family members wash their hands with soap after defecating, and before eating or preparing food.

Having all family members use a latrine.

Quickly disposing of the stool of a young child by putting it into a latrine or by burying it.

TREATMENT PLAN B
TO TREAT DEHYDRATION

1. AMOUNT OF ORS SOLUTION TO GIVE IN FIRST 4 TO 6 HOURS

Patient's age	2 4 6 8 10 12 18 2 3 4 6 8 15 adult ├──months ──→ ←──── years ────→					
Patient's weight in kilograms	3 5 7 9 11 13 15 20 30 40 50					
Give this much solution for 4-6 hours — in ml	200-400	400-600	600-800	800-1000	1000-2000	2000-4000
in local unit of measure						

- Use the patient's age only when you do not know the weight.

NOTE: ENCOURAGE THE MOTHER TO CONTINUE BREAST-FEEDING.

If the patient wants more ORS, give more.
If the eyelids become puffy, stop ORS and give other fluids. If diarrhoea continues, use ORS again when the puffiness is gone.
If the child vomits, wait 10 minutes and then continue giving ORS, but more slowly.

2. IF THE MOTHER CAN REMAIN AT THE HEALTH CENTRE

- Show her how much solution to give her child.
- Show her how to give it — a spoonful every 1 to 2 minutes.
- Check from time to time to see if she has problems.

3. AFTER 4 TO 6 HOURS, REASSESS THE CHILD USING THE ASSESSMENT CHART. THEN CHOOSE THE SUITABLE TREATMENT PLAN.

Note: If a child will continue on Plan B, tell the mother to offer small amounts of food.

If the child is under 12 months, tell the mother to:
- continue breast-feeding or
- if she does not breast-feed, give 100-200 ml of clean water before continuing ORS.

4. IF THE MOTHER MUST LEAVE ANY TIME BEFORE COMPLETING TREATMENT PLAN B

- Give her enough ORS packets for 2 days and show her how to prepare the fluid.
- Show her how much ORS to give to finish the 4-6 hour treatment at home.
- Tell her to give the child as much ORS and other fluids as he or she wants after the 4-6 hour treatment is finished.
- Tell her to offer the child small amounts of food every 3-4 hours.
- Tell her to bring the child back to the health worker if the child has any of the following:
  - passes many stools ⎫
  - is very thirsty ⎬ These 3 signs suggest the child is dehydrated.
  - has sunken eyes ⎭
  - has a fever
  - does not eat or drink normally
  - seems not to be getting better.

TREATMENT PLAN C
TO TREAT SEVERE
DEHYDRATION QUICKLY

Follow the arrows. If the answer to the questions is 'yes', go across. If it is 'no', go down.

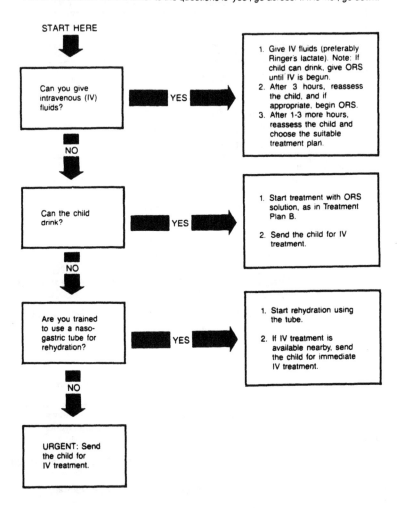

START HERE

Can you give intravenous (IV) fluids?

YES

1. Give IV fluids (preferably Ringer's lactate). Note: If child can drink, give ORS until IV is begun.
2. After 3 hours, reassess the child, and if appropriate, begin ORS.
3. After 1-3 more hours, reassess the child and choose the suitable treatment plan.

NO

Can the child drink?

YES

1. Start treatment with ORS solution, as in Treatment Plan B.

2. Send the child for IV treatment.

NO

Are you trained to use a naso-gastric tube for rehydration?

YES

1. Start rehydration using the tube.

2. If IV treatment is available nearby, send the child for immediate IV treatment.

NO

URGENT: Send the child for IV treatment.

NOTE: If the child is above 2 years of age and cholera is known to be currently occurring in your area, suspect cholera and give an appropriate oral antibiotic once the child is alert.

Antimicrobial agents used in the treatment of specific causes of diarrhoea

Cause	Antibiotic(s) of choice[1]	Alternative(s)[1]
Cholera[2,3]	**Tetracycline** Children: 12.5 mg/kg 4 times a day x 3 days Adults: 500 mg 4 times a day x 3 days *or* **Doxycycline** Adults: 300 mg once	**Furazolidone** Children: 1.25 mg/kg 4 times a day x 3 days Adults: 100 mg 4 times a day x 3 days *or* **Trimethoprim (TMP)-Sulfamethoxazole (SMX)[4]** Children: TMP 5 mg/kg and SMX 25 mg/kg twice a day x 3 days Adults: TMP 160 mg and SMX 800 mg twice a day x 3 days
Shigella dysentery[2]	**Trimethoprim (TMP)-Sulfamethoxazole (SMX)** Children: TMP 5 mg/kg and SMX 25 mg/kg twice a day x 5 days Adults: TMP 160 mg and SMX 800 mg twice a day x 5 days	**Nalidixic Acid** Children: 15 mg/kg 4 times a day x 5 days Adults: 1 g 3 times a day x 5 days *or* **Ampicillin** Children: 25 mg/kg 4 times a day x 5 days Adults: 1 g 4 times a day x 5 days
Amoebiasis	**Metronidazole** Children: 10 mg/kg 3 times a day x 5 days (10 days for severe disease) Adults: 750 mg 3 times a day x 5 days (10 days for severe disease)	In very severe cases: Dehydroemetine hydrochloride by deep, intramuscular injection, 1-1.5 mg/kg daily (maximum 90 mg) for up to 5 days, depending on response (all ages)
Giardiasis	**Metronidazole[5]** Children: 5 mg/kg 3 times a day x 5 days Adults: 250 mg 3 times a day x 5 days	**Quinacrine** Children: 2.5 mg/kg 3 times a day x 5 days Adults: 100 mg 3 times a day x 5 days

[1] All doses shown are for oral administration unless otherwise indicated. If drugs are not available in liquid form for use in young children, it may be necessary to approximate the doses given in this table.

[2] The choice of antibiotic will depend on the frequency of resistance to antibiotics in the area.

[3] Antibiotic therapy is not essential for successful treatment, but it shortens the duration of illness and the period of excretion of organisms in severe cases.

[4] Other alternatives are erythromycin and chloramphenicol.

[5] Tinidazole and ornidazole can also be used in accordance with the manufacturers' recommendations.

Treatment of fever

DIAGNOSIS / SYMPTOM \ AGE / WEIGHT		4 kg — 2 months	8 kg — 1 year	15 kg — 5 years	35 kg — 15 years / ADULT
Fever in mal-nourished or poor condition patient or when in doubt		Refer			
Fever with chills assuming it is malaria	Refer	Chloroquine (2) tab 150mg base ½ tab at once, then ¼ tab. after 6h, 24h and 48h	Chloroquine (2) tab 150mg base 1 tab at once, then ½ tab. after 6h, 24h and 48h	Chloroquine (2) tab 150mg base 2 tab at once, then 1 tab. after 6h, 24h and 48h	Chloroquine (2) tab 150mg base 4 tab at once, then 2 tab. after 6 h, 24h and 48 h
Fever with cough	Refer	See "Respiratory tract infection"			
Fever (unspecified)	Refer	Paracetamol tab 100 mg ½ tab. x 3 for 1 to 3 days	Paracetamol tab 100 mg 1 tab. x 3 for 1 to 3 days	ASA tab 300 mg 1 tab. x 3 for 1 to 3 days	ASA tab 300 mg 2 tab. x 3 for 1 to 3 days

(2) *Chloroquine 150 mg base is equivalent to 250 mg chloroquine phosphate or to 200 mg chloroquine sulfate*

Note: chloroquine is effective for malaria vivax, ovale, and malariae. However, falciparum malaria shows increasing drug-resistance. The following are examples of treatment regimens in cases of **chloroquine-resistant falciparum malaria**:

Medication	Regimen
quinine	30mg/kg/day in 3 doses for 7 days
+ tetracycline	1500mg/day in 3 doses for 7 days
sulfadoxine-pyramethamine (Fansidar)	3 tabs (25mg + 500mg) stat
mefloquine	1.0–1.5g in 2 doses 6-8hrs apart

Treatment of acute respiratory infections

DIAGNOSIS SYMPTOM \ AGE / WEIGHT		4 kg / 2 months	8 kg / 1 year	15 kg / 5 years	35 kg / 15 years	ADULT
Severe pneumonia Annex 3		Give the first dose of cotrimoxazole (see pneumonia) and **refer**				
Pneumonia Annex 3	**Refer**	Cotrimoxazole tab 400 mg SMX + 80 mg TMP ½ tab. x 2 for 5 days	Cotrimoxazole tab 400 mg SMX + 80 mg TMP 1 tab. x 2 for 5 days	Cotrimoxazole tab 400 mg SMX + 80 mg TMP 1 tab. x 2 for 5 days	Cotrimoxazole tab 400 mg SMX + 80 mg TMP 2 tab. x 2 for 5 days	
		Reassess after 2 days; continue (breast) feeding, give fluids, clear the nose; return if breathing becomes faster or more difficult, or not able to drink or when the condition deteriorates				
No pneumonia: cough or cold Annex 3	**Refer**	Paracetamol [1] tab 100 mg ½ tab. x 3 for 3 days	Paracetamol [1] tab 100 mg ½ tab. x 3 for 3 days	ASA [1] tab 300 mg 1 tab. x 3 for 3 days	ASA [1] tab 300 mg 2 tab. x 3 for 3 days	
		Supportive therapy; continue (breast) feeding, give fluids, clear the nose; return if breathing becomes faster or more difficult, or not able to drink or condition deteriorates				
Prolonged cough (over 30 days)		**Refer**				
Acute ear pain and/or ear discharge For **less** than 2 weeks	**Refer**	Cotrimoxazole tab 400 mg SMX + 80 mg TMP ½ tab. x 2 for 5 days [1]	Cotrimoxazole tab 400 mg SMX + 80 mg TMP ½ tab. x 2 for 5 days [1]	Cotrimoxazole tab 400 mg SMX + 80 mg TMP ½ tab. x 2 for 5 days	Cotrimoxazole tab 400 mg SMX + 80 mg TMP ½ tab. x 2 for 5 days	
Ear discharge For **more** than 2 weeks, no pain or fever		Clean the ear once daily by syringe without needle using lukewarm clean water. Repeat until the water comes out clean. Dry repeatedly with clean piece of cloth.				

(1) *If fever is present*

Appendix 9: Vaccine storage, immunisation schedules, drug storage.

(TT – tetanus toxoid)
(DPT– diptheria, pertussis, tetanus, also called 'triple vaccine')
(OPV– oral polio vaccine)

Vaccine storage

In a health centre, vaccines must be stored in a refrigerator at a temperature between 0–8° C. DPT and TT are damaged by freezing. OPV, measles and BCG are not; they can be frozen and refrozen without damage. Expired vaccines, and vaccines damaged by freezing or a breakdown in the cold chain, must be thrown away. Vials containing partially used, reconstituted vaccine (measles, BCG) must be thrown away after one immunisation session.

Immunisation schedules

Children

Measles: normally at 9 months, but during outbreaks and/or emergency phase at 6 months with a repeat at 9 months

BCG: at birth

DPT: dose 1 at 6 weeks
          dose 2 at 10 weeks
          dose 3 at 14 weeks

Polio: dose 1 at birth
          dose 2 at 6 weeks
          dose 3 at 10 weeks
          dose 4 at 14 weeks

TT for women of reproductive age

TT1: at first contact or as early as possible during the pregnancy

TT2: 4 weeks after TT1

TT3: 6 to 12 months after TT2 or during next pregnancy

TT4: 1 to 3 years after TT3 or during next pregnancy

TT5: 1 to 5 years after TT4 or during next pregnancy

Drug storage — practical points

- Make sure all instructions for use are clearly written in a locally understood language.
- All external containers should be clearly marked to facilitate sorting and storage.
- Packaging should be robust and weather-proof.
- All drugs supplied should have a remaining shelf-life of at least six months, with the expiry date printed on the outer carton.
- Ensure cool and dry storage room(s).
- Establish strict inventory controls.
- Ensure systematic monitoring of requisitions.

Appendix 10

Sample monitoring and surveillance form — mortality

Site_____From___/___/___To___/___/___

1. Poplulation

a. Total population at beginning of week_____

b. Births_____Deaths_____

c. Arrivals____Departures_____

d. Total population at the end of the week:_____

e. Total population <5years of age_____

2. Mortality

Reported cause of death	0–4 years Males	0–4 years Females	5+ years Males	5+ years Females	Total
Diarrhoeal disease					
Respiratory disease					
Malnutrition					
Measles					
Malaria					
Other/unknown					
Total <5 years			XXXX	XXXX	
Grand total					

Average total mortality rate_____
(Deaths/10,000 total population/day average for week

Average under-five mortality rate_____
(Deaths/10,000 under fives/day average for week

Sample monitoring and surveillance form — morbidity

Primary symptoms /diagnosis	0–4 years Males	0–4 years Females	5+ years Males	5+ years Females	Total
Watery diarrhoea/ dehydration					
Bloody diarrhoea					
Fever with cough					
Fever & chills/ Malaria					
Measles					
Suspected hepatitis					
Suspected cholera					
Suspected meningitis					
Other/unknown					
Total					

Notes

1. It is essential that clear case-definitions are agreed by all medical staff and supervision includes checking of definitions.

2. It is also essential to agree what constitutes a 'new case' and which is the primary diagnosis where a patient presents with two complaints e.g. cough and diarrhoea.

References and further reading

Benenson A S (ed) (1990), *Control of Communicable Diseases in Man*, New York: American Public Health Association.

Cairncross S, Feachem R G (1983), *Environmental Health Engineering in the Tropics:An Introductory Text*. New York.: Wiley.

Centers for Disease Control (CDC) (1992), *Famine–affected, Refugee and Displaced Populations: Recommendations for Public Health Issues*, Morbidity and Mortality Weekly Report 41 (No.RR–13), Atlanta, Georgia: CDC.

CDC (1992), *Guidelines for Collecting, Processing, Storing, and Shipping Diagnostic Specimens in Refugee Health–care Environments* (Annex A, supplement to MMWR report no.41), Atlanta: CDC.

Crofton J, Horne N, and Miller F (1992), *Clinical Tuberculosis*, London: Macmillan and TALC.

Johns W (1987), *Establishing a Refugee Camp Laboratory*, London: SCF.

Lusty T and Diskett P (1984), *Selective Feeding Programmes*, Oxfam Practical Health Guide No.1, Oxford: Oxfam.

Medecins sans Frontieres (1988), *Clinical Guidelines, Diagnostic and Treatment Manual*, Paris: Hatier.

NGO Working Group on Refugee Women (1989), *Working with Women: A Practical Guide*, Geneva.

Sandler, R and Jones, T C (1987) *Medical Care of Refugees*, Oxford: Oxford University Press.

Simmonds et al (1985) *Refugee Community Health Care*, Oxford: Oxford University Press

Thomson M, (forthcoming) Disease vector control in refugee camps, Oxford: Oxfam.

Tropical Doctor (1991), 21, supplement 1, Disasters.

UNHCR (1982), *Handbook for Emergencies*, Geneva: UNHCR.

UNHCR (1992), *Water Manual for Refugee Situations*. Geneva: UNHCR.

UNICEF (1986), *Assisting in Emergencies:A Resource Handbook for UNICEF Field Staff*, New York: UNICEF.

Werner D, (1982), *Helping Health Workers Learn*, Hesperian Foundation.

World Health Organisation (WHO) (1983), *Measuring Change in Nutritional Status*, Geneva: WHO (currently under revision).

(WHO) (1989), *Immunisation in Practice*, Oxford and Geneva, Oxford University Press and WHO.

WHO (1990), *A Manual for the Treatment of Diarrhoea*, Geneva:WHO.

WHO (1992), *The Use of Essential Drugs*, Geneva:WHO.

WHO (1992), *Guidelines forCholera Control*, Geneva:WHO

WHO (undated), *The New Emergency Health Kit*, Geneva:WHO.

Young H (1992), *Food Scarcity and Famine: Assessment and Res*ponse, Oxfam Practical Health Guide No.7, Oxford: Oxfam.

Glossary

Assessment: A process which may or may not be systematic, of gathering information, analysing it and then making a judgement on the basis of it.

Attack rate (see incidence rate)

Case fatality rate (see mortality rate).

Chemoprophylaxis: The administration of a chemical, including antibiotics, to prevent the development of an infection or the progression of an infection to clinical disease.

Communicable disease: Illness which is caused by a specific infectious agent or its toxic products, and which arises through transmission of that agent or its products from a reservoir to a susceptible host.

Community health worker: A person selected and trained to provide certain kinds of health care to a community, usually preventive and basic curative care. May work only from home or also from a small health post, and the work usually involves home visiting.

Coverage: The extent to which those who need a service are actually receiving it (e.g. the proportion of pregnant women receiving ante–natal care in a given catchment area).

Demographic data: Data which describes a population by age, sex, birth rates, death rates etc.

Epidemiology: The study of the distribution and determinants of disease frequency in human populations.

Incidence rate: A measure of the frequency of cases of disease in a particular population, the times of onset of which occured during a specified period of time. Incidence rates which are calculated for narrowly defined populations (in terms of age, sex, etc) during intervals of time, as in epidemics, are often called **attack rates**.

Indicator: Something which provides a basis for measuring progress towards objectives. It may relate to quantitative or qualitative factors, and acts as a 'marker'0 to show what progress has been made to date.

Morbidity: The state of being diseased.

Mortality (death) rate: A measure of the frequency of deaths within a particular population during a specified interval of time. If deaths from all causes are included, the rate is called a **crude mortality rate**. If only deaths from a specified cause are included, the rate is called a **cause–specific mortality rate**.
A **case fatality rate** is a measure of the frequency of deaths due to a particular disease among members of a population who have the disease (i.e.cases).

Prevalence rate: A measure of the frequency of all current cases of a disease (regardless of the time of onset) within a particular population, either at a specified instant (point–prevalence rate) or during a specified period (period–prevalence rate).

Qualitative: Qualitative information is that which may be used to describe relationships between points of interest, such as malnutrition and various causal factors.

Quantitative: Quantitative information is used to measure the degree to which some feature of interest is present such as the prevalence of malnutrition.

Random sample: A method of selecting members of a population in such a way that everyone has an equal chance of being selected.

Risk factor : A factor which increases the chances of a person developing a disease or a problem.

Screening : A fast way to identify people with risk factors or the first symptoms of a specific disease.

Surveillance of disease: The continuing scrutiny of all those aspects of the occurrence and spread of disease that are pertinent to effective control.

Task analysis: A systematic way of looking at work which is being performed in relation to a specific purpose.

Transmission: The direct (contact or droplet spread) or indirect (vectorborne, vehicle–borne, airborne) transfer of an infectious agent from a reservoir to a susceptible host.

Triage: To sort patients into groups according to severity of illness so that priorities can be established to use available facilities most effectively and efficiently. Where facilities are limited and needs are many and urgent, difficult decisions may have to be made "to do the best for the most".

Vector: An animal, frequently an arthropod, which transfers an infectious agent from a source of infection to a susceptible host.

Index

access, to services in the camp 15
acute lower respiratory tract infections 35
AIDS 31, 37-8
amoebiasis 97
anaemia 9, 22, 50, 76, 80
ancillary workers 40, 46
anthropometric measurements (children) 61-73
assessment 3-13, 106
  for evaluation 54-5
  medical problems 93
attack rates 106
auxiliary staff *see* ancillary workers

BCG vaccinations 37
beriberi 50, 79
birth attendants, traditional 40, 41-2
biscuits (Food Aid) 21, 75
body measurements (children) 61-73
breastfeeding 22, 94, 95

camp environment 5-6
case fatality rate 106, 107
chemoprophylaxis 106
children:
  body measurements 61-73
  feeding programmes 21, 22-3
  health care 41-2, 76
  and sanitation 9, 27, 94
chlorination (water) 25-6, 87
chloroquine-resistant malaria, treatment for 34, 98
cholera:
  control 33-4

treatment for 96, 97
clinical care 38-43
  in the camp 11-12
  disease treatment protocols 92-9
  and long-term displacement 52
cold chains (immunisation) 30
colds, treatment for 99
communicable diseases 11, 31-8, 106
communications 6
community health workers 40, 46, 106
control, of diseases 31-8
co-ordination, of services 14
corn soya milk, porridge recipe 85
cough, treatment for 99
coverage (services) 106
cretinism 81
crude mortality rates 59-60, 107

data collection:
  for evaluation 56
  for Health Information System 17-18
death *see* mortality
deforestation 49
dehydration 93, 95-6
demographic data 106
demography 5
diarrhoea 76, 93
  antimicrobial treatment for 97
  control 33-4
  treatment for 94
disability 4, 15, 44, 51-2
disadvantaged groups *see* vulnerable groups
diseases:
  assessment information 11

control 15, 31-8, 51
surveillance 107
treatment protocols 92-9
vector-borne *see* names of specific diseases; vectors
displacement, long-term 48-53
distribution (food) 21-2, 23
drainage, in camp 8
dried skimmed milk, porridge recipe 84-5
drugs:
essential 12, 42-3, 88-91
storage 101
dry distribution (food) 21-2
dysentery 11, 93
control 34
treatment for 97

ear pain/discharge, treatment for 99
ecological impact, of long-term displacement 49
elderly 4, 15
Emergency Health Kit 43, 88-99
environmental health 7-9, 24-9, 50
epidemics 32-3
epidemiology 106
equity, in the camp 15
evaluation 54-7
excreta, disposal 8, 9, 26, 27

faeces *see* excreta
feeding *see* selective feeding; supplementary feeding;
therapeutic feeding
fever 93, 98
folic acid deficiency 76, 80
food:
availability 9-10
distribution 21-2, 23
nutritional values 74-5
see also rations
food basket *see* general ration

general ration 10, 19-20, 23
giardiasis, treatment for 97

goitre 81
guidelines, standardisation 13-14

handwashing 8, 9, 94
healers 40, 46
health, environmental see environmental health
health care, preventive measures 15, 24-31
health centres:
facilities 38-9
organisation 39
staffing 40
health coordinator 40
Health Information System 17-18, 49, 51
health promotion campaigns 31, 51
health status:
in the camp, assessment 11
newcomer screening 48
health supplies 39, 88-91
health workers 12, 40, 45-7, 52-3
hepatitis 35
high energy milk (recipe) 86
HIV 29, 31, 37-8
host community, good relations with 15-16, 39
hygiene promotion 9, 26

immunisation 29-31, 33, 51
in the camp 12
schedules 100-1
incidence rate 106
indicators 55-6, 107
information *see* assessment; data collection;
qualitative/quantative information
integration, of services 14
iodine deficiency 81
iron-deficiency anaemia *see* anaemia

laboratory facilities 42
laboratory technician 40, 42
latrines 8, 26-7, 94

literacy training 53
logistics 6, 15
long-term displacement 48-53

malaria 11, 27
  control 34-5
  treatment for 98
malnutrition, surveys 9, 11, 18-19, 61
malted grain porridge 82-3
measles 11, 29, 33, 35, 76, 77, 79
measurements, for nutrition surveys 61-73
medical care *see* clinical care
medical supplies 88-91
meningitis 30, 35-6
meningococcal meningitis 30, 35-6
midwives 40-2
milk *see* dried skimmed milk; high energy milk
mineral deficiences 11, 50, 76-81
minority groups 15, 44
money, in camp 6
monitoring and surveillance:
  clinical care 40
  diseases 107
  environmental health 28-9
  immunisation 30
  morbidity 11
  nutrition 23
  psycho-social issues 45
  sample forms 102-3
  women and children health care 42
morbidity 11, 103
mortality 11, 102
mortality rates 59-60, 107
mother-and-child-health services 40-2

niacin deficiency 80
nutrition:
  monitoring, and long-term displacement 49-50
  screening 23
  status, in camp 9, 18-19
  surveillance 23
  surveys 9, 18-19, 61-73

oral rehydration therapy 12

participation:
  for evaluation 56
  of refugees 14, 26
pellagra 76, 80
planning 13-16
pneumonia 35, 99
pollution, water supply 7-8, 25, 26
porridge recipes 82-5
post-traumatic stress disorder 45
pregnancy 41-2
prevalence rate 107
prevention, health care 15, 24-31
psycho-social issues:
  in the camp 12-13, 43-5
  and long-term displacement 52

qualitative/quantative information 56, 107

random sample 107
rations:
  general ration 10, 19-20, 23
  and long-term displacement 50
recipes, supplementary feeding 82-6
referral facilities, for health care 16, 39
rehabilitation 44
resources, and planning 15
respiratory tract infections 35, 76, 99
risk factors 11, 107
rubbish, disposal 8

sampling, for nutrition survey 61-2
sanitation:
  in camp 8-9, 26-7, 40
  emergency, and long-term displacement 49
screening 23, 107
scurvy 50, 76, 79
selective feeding 10-11
services, in the camp 14-15
shelter 7, 29, 49
shigellosis 34, 93, 97

solid waste, disposal 8, 27
staffing, of camp 6
    see also health workers
STDs 31, 38
storage facilities 6, 100-1
supplementary feeding 10-11, 20-2, 23, 50
    recipes 82-6
surveillance *see* monitoring and surveillance
surveys *see* malnutrition surveys; nutrition surveys

task analysis 107
temporary structures, and long-term displacement 49
therapeutic feeding 10-11, 22-3
thiamine deficiency 50, 79
traditional birth attendants 40, 41-2
training 45-7
    and long-term displacement 52-3
    and psycho-social issues 44-5
    women 40, 46
transmission 108
transport 6
treatment protocols, for diseases 92-9
triage 12, 39, 108
tuberculosis 29, 36-7, 38

undernutrition 93

vaccination 29, 37
vaccine storage 100
vectors and vector-borne diseases 108
    control 8-9, 27-9, 34
    and long-term displacement 49
vitamin A:
    deficiency 9, 29-30, 50, 76, 77-9
    and measles 33
vitamin B deficiency 9
vitamin C deficiency 9, 50, 76, 79
vitamin deficiences 11, 50, 76-81
vulnerable groups 4
    access to health services 15
    assessment information 11

and long-term displacement 48
psycho-social issues 43-4
supplementary feeding 20, 21

washing facilities 8
waste disposal 8, 9, 26, 27
waste water, disposal 27
water:
    carrying 25
    quality 24-5, 87
    quantities required 7, 24-5
    storage 8, 26
    testing 8, 87
    treatment 25-6
    trucking/tankering 25
water supply:
    in camp 7-8, 24-6
    chlorination 25-6, 87
    and long-term displacement 49
    pollution 7-8, 25, 26
    and vector control 28
wet distribution (food) 21-2
women:
    and deforestation 49
    health care 4, 11, 39, 41-2
    literacy teaching 53
    participation in planning 14, 26
    privacy needs 8, 27, 39
    psycho-social issues 44, 52
    sanitary materials 27
    training 40

xeropthalmia 29, 76, 77-9